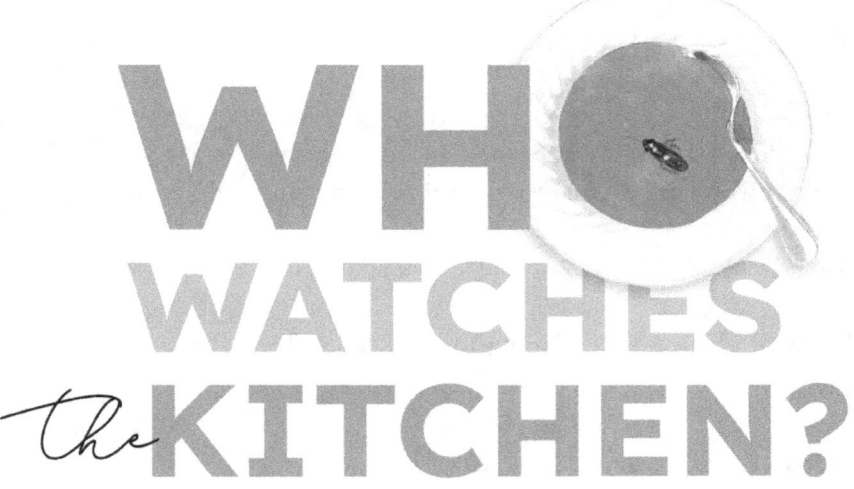

WHO WATCHES *the* KITCHEN?

A HEALTH INSPECTOR UNCOVERS THE DIRT ON HER WAY TO SAFE FOOD ADVOCACY

Francine L. Shaw, CP-FS. FMP.

Cover Design and Illustrations: Amber E. Buhrman
Interior Design and Formatting: Toni Serofin, Sanserofin Studio

ISBN 979-8-9864073-0-2

Library of Congress Cataloging-in-Publication Data available upon request.

Printed in the United States of America

Second Edition

I want to dedicate this book to my "Aunt Pat" who, without even realizing it, showed me there was a different lifestyle than the one I was living. Because of her, I knew there was a light at the end of the tunnel, and if I worked hard enough, one day I would see it.

Contents

Foreword

W hen I ask restaurant operators if they are having or have had any food safety issues in their restaurants, one of the most common statements I hear is: "We haven't had any outbreaks that I can remember so, no, we don't have any food safety issues."

I follow up by asking if they've had customer complaints of illness, allergy, or injury from physical hazards in the last month, social media reports of illness from several customers in the last month, or a health department inspection initiated due to reports of customer illnesses. I ask if they've gotten a low grade or score on the most current health inspection report or had any critical violations of Foodborne Illness Risk Factors, which are the strongest bellwethers of risk. By the time I'm done asking, they often reluctantly acknowledge that they might actually have had a food safety issue in the past.

Many restaurant operators don't associate day-to-day food safety compliance issues in their operations with a customer's foodborne illness risk unless they experience a foodborne illness outbreak—or afterward, when they have already caused a foodborne disease outbreak. However, based on numerous studies by the US Food and Drug Administration (FDA), Centers for Disease Control and Prevention (CDC), and state public health experts, a restaurant is more likely to cause a single sporadic case of foodborne illness, in a single location, than to experience a foodborne disease outbreak in which two or more people get sick from the same contaminated food.

In support of these observations, the Interagency Food Safety Analytics Collaboration (IFSAC), a forum of CDC, FDA, and US

Department of Agriculture (USDA) experts, has shown that there can be significantly more sporadic cases of foodborne disease caused by the bacterial pathogens *Campylobacter*, *E. coli* O157, *Listeria monocytogenes*, and *Salmonella* each year than outbreak-associated cases caused by these same pathogens.[1] For example, a study of foodborne illnesses in the United States analyzed by IFSAC using FoodNet data (representing only 15 percent of the US population) identified 195 cases of *Campylobacter* illness associated with outbreaks between 2004 and 2011; by contrast, there were 42,744 single, sporadic cases of the same illness during this same time period.

Foodborne disease outbreaks caused by foods prepared and sold in foodservice establishments (i.e., restaurants and any other retail foodservice businesses that prepare food for immediate consumption and sell it directly to a consumer) continue to be a major public health issue in the United States. The CDC states that over 64 percent of the foodborne disease outbreaks that occurred in 2017 in the United States were linked to restaurants (the average is closer to 60 percent per year). Interestingly, the largest percentage of foodborne disease outbreaks caused by restaurants in 2017 came from sit-down dining restaurants, not fast-food or quick-serve restaurants (and this is similar year to year).[2]

Customers are also more aware of a food safety risk at restaurants now than they were before the COVID-19 pandemic. Fully 74 percent of consumers state that it is somewhat or very common to get food poisoning from restaurants.[3] Safety is the top priority for choosing

---

[1] Ebel, Eric D., Michael S. Williams, Dana Cole, Curtis C. Travis, Karl C. Klontz, Neal J. Golden, and Robert M. Hoekstra. "Comparing Characteristics of Sporadic and Outbreak-Associated Foodborne Illnesses, United States, 2004–2011." Emerging Infectious Diseases 22, no. 7 (2016): 1193-1200. https://doi.org/10.3201/eid2207.150833.

[2] Centers for Disease Control and Prevention. "Burden of Foodborne Illness: Findings." Last reviewed: November 5, 2018. https://www.cdc.gov/foodborneburden/2011-foodborne-estimates.html.

[3] U.S. Food & Drug Administration. "FDA Releases Food Safety and Nutrition Survey Results." Last updated November 9, 2021. https://www.fda.gov/food/cfsan-constituent-updates/fda-releases-food-safety-and-nutrition-survey-results.

which restaurant to patronize,[4] and customers say they plan to spend twice as much per month with restaurants that meet cleaning and safety standards.[5]

Well, we have heard from many authorities about the outcomes of food safety risk in restaurants, including government and industry experts, but rarely do we have an opportunity to hear about what actually goes on inside a restaurant kitchen that results in the restaurant *causing* a foodborne illness or outbreak. Now we do, and from a foodservice business leader and operator who actually managed and grew a very successful independent restaurant business for twenty years and who also just so happens to be a former health department inspector.

In this book, *Who Watches the Kitchen: A Health Inspector Uncovers the Dirt on Her Way to Safe Food Advocacy,* Francine gives us this important perspective. It's a perspective consumers need to hear. It's also a perspective we stakeholders in the restaurant industry need to hear if we are going to reduce food safety risks. So many poor business decisions are a contributing factor to foodborne illness and disease; this book opens our eyes and helps us avoid these risky choices.

A single independent restaurant operator or a restaurant enterprise (sometimes referred to as a restaurant chain or franchise business, with multiple restaurant locations) can have all the best-in-class standard operating procedures (SOPs), training materials, cleaning and sanitation plans and chemicals, equipment, and restaurant facility design. But when one employee or manager decides not to follow basic personal hygiene or these extensive plans, someone is going to get a foodborne illness.

Francine gets right to the point, describing these events by managers and employees from her earliest experiences as a restaurant employee

---

[4] CSSI Marketing + Culinary. "Datassential's One Table Consumer Report: 5 Takeaways." Posted July 24, 2020. https://www.cssiculinary.com/datassentials-one-table-consumer-report-5-takeaways.

[5] Simon-Kucher. "Recent Study Reveals that Restaurants' Sanitation Standards Now Influence Consumer Purchase Behavior More Than Price of Menu Items." Posted March 9, 2021. https://www.simon-kucher.com/en/who-we-are/newsroom/recent-study-reveals-restaurants-sanitation-standards-now-influence-consumer.

to her observations as a health inspector in thousands of restaurants over the course of her career.

Francine describes her early career working for a manager who refused to discard ice cream mix that had cockroaches in it, intending to reduce food waste and avoid the extra cost of replacing the mix, and another who had two sets of SOPs to prepare food—one for daily use, and one for when the local health inspector made a visit.

Francine writes that many restaurants likely do not get health inspections on a regular basis, and some managers are shocked when there is an unannounced inspection they feel they are unprepared for and demand to be alerted before an inspection. Another restaurant brand she inspected, one Francine patronized as a customer, seemed nice in the dining room, but the kitchen she describes was a nightmare of dirty storage containers holding old food, dirty storage racks, open food stored on the floor, dirty dishware, and cockroaches all over the place even in the daylight.

...if you're a fellow industry professional, this book will be insightful for developing your training plans...

I won't share all the other stories here and "spoil" the ending of the book, so keep reading and take notes. If you're a restaurant patron, you'll come to know what to look for in choosing where to eat and keeping your own kitchen safe. And if you're a fellow industry professional, this book will be insightful for developing your training plans, how you measure employee and manager compliance with your requirements, and how you execute your performance rating process to weed out non-compliant employees.

Finally, Francine writes with the intention to share her experiences to help other food safety professionals (all of us) get better. She has turned her knowledge and experience into thought leadership that is beneficial to the entire foodservice and sales industry.

Restaurant consumers may also find this book helpful in finding out what is really going on in some of their favorite restaurant kitchens, and in learning just how important health inspections are to their public health. However, Francine doesn't just tell the bad stories, but also the good ones. She has turned this knowledge into several successful businesses that support, advise, and enable the food industry to reduce food safety risk—something very few attempt to do and accomplish so well—making her a valued public health professional to our nation.

Hal King, Ph.D.
Managing Partner, Active Food Safety LLC

Preface

Many excellent books about the foodservice industry are available. Several of them are written by friends of mine for whom I have a great deal of respect.

Over the years, though, I have searched for books other than celebrity chef memoirs that tell the behind-the-scenes stories of life in the industry, and I've found it difficult to find any. Yet you can sit down to lunch with industry folks like me and hear a multitude of scenarios that are less than appetizing. If you have a weak stomach, we may not be the best group of individuals to dine with.

I am frequently asked, "What is the worst thing you've ever seen?" The answer to that question depends on what portion of my career you're referring to. I have had many horrid food safety experiences. I have worked in restaurants as an employee and manager and have conducted training and education for the foodservice industry. I've undertaken third-party inspections, which are sometimes announced before they happen and therefore give the establishment time to prepare, and health inspections, which are always unannounced.

I've done both corporate training and public training on food safety and heard grim tales during both. The stories people will share are nothing short of shocking, and sometimes incredibly sad. For example, I had a lady share that she lost her child in the third trimester of a pregnancy due to a foodborne illness she contracted at a restaurant. These training days remind me why I am in the food safety business.

I've also taught many classes for local colleges. It has felt good to make an impression on the young folks and their attitudes toward food safety. Many of these students hadn't been taught the basics at home, or they had severe misconceptions.

I share these food safety stories to help others understand what it is like to work behind the scenes in the foodservice industry and to give an honest snapshot of what it was like to be a health inspector—no fluff. These are the stories that no one prepares you for, and you don't learn them from a textbook in a university. I also write to let other women know how far we have come in achieving gender equality in this space in the last ten, twenty, thirty years.

I have always believed that life should be fun regardless of what you do. Learning is more effective, and people learn more, if it is fun. Employees are also more productive. Fun is how I have tried to approach most of my adult life. When I started my own company, the brand colors I chose were intentionally bright pink and bright green—fun, bright, distinctive.

Entrepreneurship is a far cry from where I began, and it was quite a journey to get here. As you will see in my story, some aspects are very personal. Nothing happens overnight, but with hard work, persistence, and belief in yourself, you can get wherever you want to go. I hope my story provides someone with the inspiration and courage they need to believe in themself enough to do something they thought was impossible.

I offer tidbits of education, funny stories, scenarios where I thought I would lose my mind, others where I thought my heart would break, and an occasion or two when I honestly thought I might die. I hope you enjoy reading the book as much as I did writing it.

Prologue

During my formative years in the foodservice industry, I worked with many people. Some were excellent leaders, others not so much. Both kinds provided me with a plethora of knowledge; I was like a sponge, and I learned from everyone.

I learned how to treat people with kindness and respect. I observed good leaders asking their team members to do things that needed to be done rather than barking orders. I saw one leader throw a travel bag at an employee when the employee could not find someone to replace a sick contractor. (Mental note: Don't ever do this.)

Learning how to correct behavior without demeaning an individual is one of a leader's most valuable lessons. There is never a need to make another human being feel insignificant. I spent years observing others and learning. I'm still learning. I believe we should learn something new every day.

Over time, I've seen some less-than-appetizing sights, but they were rare, typically isolated to those less-than-excellent leaders. I remember working in one unit where the manager would eat food on the prep line. Bacon wrapped in swiss cheese, dipped in mushroom sauce, was his go-to. He would stand at the end of the prep table for the entire lunch rush, dipping and eating (mouth open), snapping orders at the crew. The whole scene was simply disgusting. I can still see him screaming, the spit droplets spewing from his mouth.

Eating on a line: a definite no-no.

Working at multiple facilities during my years in the business exposed me to a wide variety of food code violations. I worked with one individual who kept all of his facility's cleaning supplies in the trunk of his car. When we ran out of something, we couldn't do anything about it—until he came to work. Out of dish soap? Too bad, the manager will be in tomorrow. He also kept used mopheads in empty pickle buckets so he could wash them at home rather than purchase new ones. Sometimes they'd be in there so long, they harbored maggots.

Once, when cleaning a shake machine, I drained all of the mixes and took the lids off the top to discover cockroaches floating on top of the leftover ice milk. I nearly had a heart attack! Our state's health regulations permitted us to save the shake mix at night and reuse it the next day, as long as we broke the cycle weekly. It was my first day at this location, and I was performing a training function. My mind was racing. I was young, recently promoted, and this was my first day in a new store. Could this be a joke?!

I was young, recently promoted, and this was my first day
in a new store. Could this be a joke?!

I called back to the kid putting the mix in the cooler and told him to throw it away. But if you work in foodservice, you know food cost is near and dear to every operator's heart.

The manager said to me, "You can't throw that away. Do you know how much that stuff costs?"

I told him, "We have to throw it away. There were cockroaches in it!" The poor young man at the cooler looked at us in bewilderment. What should he do?

"Cockroaches float," the manager insisted. "There won't be any in the mix."

OMG, how do you know that? I thought, as I quickly walked back to dump out the mix.

The manager was right. There were no cockroaches in it. Apparently this was not his first experience with floating cockroaches. The next day I called a pest control company. I just knew my new boss was going to fire me. Fortunately, he didn't.

A year or so later, I thought I would lose my mind when I saw employees going through garbage bags to pull out sandwich containers and unopened condiments so they could wash and reuse them to reduce expenses. Of course, they didn't do this on a whim—no one wants to dig through the trash if they don't have to. We were normally only willing to dig through trash when someone threw their retainer in the garbage, and even then, we weren't happy about it. The general manager directed the workers to do this. The same man who kept the cleaning supplies in the trunk of his car and who told us to put dirty mopheads in a clean five-gallon pickle bucket so he could take the heads home and wash them.

It doesn't sound like a big deal. But these mopheads were laden with bacteria. We used them to wash everything from restroom floors to whatever came in on the bottom of our customers' feet, not to mention everything that had spilled on the floor over time.

The smell erupting from the bucket of mopheads waiting to be washed could cause you to vomit, and on hot summer days, you could easily find maggots squirming among the rancid strings of damp cotton. Why would anyone put this nastiness into their washing machine?

I can't imagine it saved that much money, but this is the type of behavior that corporate bonus programs of the era created at fast-food restaurants. If not created with great care, bonus programs can cause all kinds of disastrous situations, especially when managers get greedy. The company I worked for had a great bonus program. The problem was, the more profitable you were in a given year, the better you were expected to be the following year. Greed led managers to do all sorts of crazy things.

Plus, a company can only increase profitability expectations to a certain point before they become unrealistic. When they become unattainable, managers begin cheating the system to earn their bonuses. Some managers had even become accustomed to a specific lifestyle they couldn't maintain without the hefty quarterly bonuses they were used to receiving. So what was intended to be a motivational incentive program had become a massive risk to the company and to their customers' health.

I heard managers tell employees to extend the expiration dates on food products. They'd water down hand soap and dish soap to the point that you couldn't get a bubble no matter how much you tried. We workers joked that we had to use a straw broom until it was down to its last straw. It was that bad. All in the name of creating a high gross profit, and an unfathomable bottom line, so managers could earn a bonus.

And then there were the days the dreaded health inspector showed up.

The manager with the cheese-wrapped bacon had two sets of standard operating policies and procedures (SOPs): SOPs from corporate and secret SOPs that took place when no higher-ups were around. Most of the time, we followed the "secret" SOPs. When the health inspector or executive management walked in the door, corporate SOPs went into effect!

This guy was a real character, and he was the king of manipulation. There are few individuals I've known before or since who could manipulate people the way he could. He was a puppet master. Not only did he have the entire store operating precisely on two different sets of SOPs, but he had employees willingly stealing for him—literally carrying product out the back door.

When I say stealing, I am not referring to a sandwich or a meal here and there. No, I am referring to whole cases of product. They would carry out cases of eggs—360 eggs at a time—that he would feed to his horses because he said it made their coats shiny. Cases of burgers, grilled chicken, cheese, salad dressing, and more would be loaded into the trunk of his car by his favorite employees. They did this to make him happy. He would offer them free meals and tickets to the horse races where his horses raced, invite them to parties at his house, and give them more hours on the schedule. Even let them make their own schedule—a teenager's dream.

This general manager always counted the weekly and the end-of-the-month inventory, so none of this theft created an issue within the company until someone like me, who wasn't willing to be part of his shenanigans, counted the inventory and came up with massive product shortages. Then guess who took the hit? The only person that ever came up short on stock. It appeared that that individual couldn't count or had inventory control issues because this was only occurring when the manager was on vacation. No one controls me, and throughout my life this has caused problems. Having this personality means I occasionally suffer the consequences. I got in so much trouble in that store.

For eighteen months, I cried almost daily on my way to work and back home. But I refused to be a puppet. The deceptions that occurred in that restaurant were such B.S. It was a no-win situation. Sometimes the manipulation and narcissism made me feel like I was crazy. But I knew that no matter how hard this man tried, I would not let him break me. Pastor Robert Schuller said, "Tough times never last, but tough people do." There was no end in sight unless someone was willing to do something about it. So I did.

"Tough times never last, but tough people do."

I was terrified, but I called the corporate office, sharing everything I knew. I had been in this position for months. This guy was putting me in a situation that compromised my integrity daily, I hated a job I had once loved, and I thought I was losing my mind.

They transferred me out of the restaurant in about a week. After an internal investigation and surveillance, human resources terminated several members of management and crew. I was relieved for the employees who were still working there. They would finally have a better working environment. And I was a stronger person, having survived the experience myself.

Experience in my early years taught me not everyone follows the rules, and though most do a good job, there are a handful of shady people in business. You can't trust everyone, even if you want to. The operators who can't or won't operate as they should negatively impact those who do.

My time and experience in operations were more than beneficial when I moved to the other side of the fence and began conducting food safety inspections. Now I knew what to look for and where to look.

I knew what happened in the less-than-stellar kitchens as soon as the words "health inspector" were uttered within the facility's walls. And I knew that good employees often got nervous and made silly mistakes when someone in a white lab coat walked in the door.

After realizing too many places did not focus on food safety and quality assurance the way I had during my career in restaurants, I transitioned to the training and education side of the industry and then founded a consulting firm. As a health inspector, I conducted thousands of food safety inspections. Most of them were good, but there were those days. Those days when I never wanted to walk into another kitchen again. Ever.

Sometimes it's not a matter of operators not caring to do their jobs properly. Managers end up in less than desirable situations for a number of reasons. When they're not trained or appropriately educated, they don't understand the ramifications of their failure to follow procedures. Other times, they are simply not provided with adequate equipment and tools. There are often cultural differences and language barriers to this issue, as well. Sometimes employees' hands are tied, and they aren't permitted to make the necessary decisions to operate their facility properly.

None of this makes health code violations permissible.

People can die from a foodborne illness (aka food poisoning). According to the CDC, 3,000 Americans every year do lose their lives to it (see *Sources*). Even more staggeringly, as many as 420,000 people die globally. My job as a food safety expert is to educate as many people as possible. If I can save one person's life, I will have made a difference.

This book will take a light-hearted but very serious look at many of my experiences as a food safety inspector.

I'm Gonna Be Somebody

In my teens, the title and chorus of Gloria Gaynor's "I Will Survive" spoke directly to my heart and my will. When I was in my late twenties, Travis Tritt's country song "I'm Gonna Be Somebody" was popular. I connected with this song more than I do with most.

I grew up in a ridiculously dysfunctional family in a region people refer to as "Pennsyltucky." Until I was about seven years old, we lived what would have been considered the typical middle-class family life. Shortly after, my parents divorced, and life as I knew it changed forever. I went from being in a middle-class family with a dad and a stay-at-home mom to being a welfare kid with a single mom who was waitressing in a bar. At the age of nine, I became responsible for my three siblings.

Kids made fun of my clothes as I walked down the hall…

We were poor, and I was reminded of it every day in school, for my entire way through school. The free lunch tickets for poor kids were a different color than the tickets the other kids bought, making my poverty evident to everyone, so I stopped eating lunch in seventh grade. Kids made fun of my clothes as I walked down the hall, and my glasses, purchased with welfare funds, weren't the latest fashion trend.

I wasn't allowed to hang out with the one or two friends I did have. I had to stay home to clean house and take care of my siblings.

I never went to a prom or even a high school dance. I had stringy (as my mother referred to it) blonde hair, large eyes, and buck teeth that stuck out so far my lips couldn't touch. I was the ugly one, and reminded of it daily. All of these things set me apart, isolated.

At twelve, I got my first paying job through a hire-a-teen advertisement I heard on local radio station W-E-E-O, WEEO. A family that owned a local insurance company hired me to babysit two days a week, to clean house and cook dinner for them. I loved this family environment. It was something I had not experienced since I was six or seven years old. Even though I was essentially their housekeeper and nanny, I still relished the atmosphere. It was an escape.

At the same time, I picked up another cleaning job through the same program. And the following summer, at thirteen, I applied for a job through a summer program for disadvantaged children. I spent that summer working at the local college, mowing grass, trimming weeds, cleaning dorms and the library. I remember cleaning the lawn around the college president's house, thinking what a beautiful home it was and dreaming that I would live in a beautiful home one day.

I hated it. Not the work. But the people I worked with, who were not kind. I preferred cleaning the dorms by myself to being in the yard with the other workers. In the yard, I could hear them making fun of me. They were as poor as I was. But they had one advantage over me—they were more attractive. I guess when you're at the proverbial bottom of society, you'll use whatever assets you have to make yourself feel better.

The following summer, I worked at the high school library. I discovered that libraries—and the Dewey decimal system—were definitely not my thing! Oh, how I despised the odor of those old books. I loved to read, but the smell of all of those books in one place was just too much.

At the beginning of tenth grade, I had an opportunity to earn a little more money. I began babysitting for five boys overnight while their mom, Mary, worked the midnight shift at Dunkin Donuts. I would stay with them through the night and then go to school during the day. These boys were a handful! They ranged in age from four to eleven years old. You'd think they'd be in bed while I was there, right? Nope. Those boys would jump out the second-floor bedroom window of the house, fistfight with one another like they were archenemies, and stage food fights with just about anything they ate—dinner, snacks, it didn't matter. They were almost uncontrollable.

Once I caught two of them outside in sub-zero temperatures, running water over their feet, trying to make themselves sick so they wouldn't have to go to school. It was like monitoring prisoners. Never a dull moment. Thank heavens for my brother's antics, or they would have terrified me. He well prepared me for these boys.

> I never enjoyed working in those conditions, but they don't freak me out like they do most people.

Mostly, though, I remember that Mary brought garbage bags full of donuts home with her in the mornings. My sisters loved it when I took donuts home for them. I also remember the cockroaches. If we didn't get the donuts out of the bag that Mary placed on top of the heater quickly enough, cockroaches would crawl in among the donuts. The house was infested with roaches, so as soon as she placed the bag on top of that warm heater, they would smell those fresh glazed donuts and move into that warm dark trash bag for their morning feast. It still gives me chills to think about it, but why wouldn't they—the smell of those donuts made your mouth water!

I have endured many cockroach experiences throughout my life, and they're all coming back to me as I write this. I wonder if those roaches in the donuts are why I never had the typical reaction to cockroach infestations as a health inspector. Don't misunderstand—I never enjoyed working in those conditions, but they don't freak me out like they do most people.

I quit that babysitting job after I was startled awake one night to find Mary's boyfriend sitting on the edge of the couch where I slept. He told me that she said it was okay if he had his way with me. I was out the door in a flash. I was fortunate that night in more ways than one. I got out of the house unharmed, and I was a fifteen-year-old girl who walked a mile home safely in the middle of the night, alone.

In December 1977, I got my first "real" job, and it was a job that changed my life forever. I lied about my age, and a manager hired me at a fast-food restaurant. When he figured out how old I was, he let me stay—I was doing a good job—but because of child labor laws he only allowed me to work at the fry station. I was the best damn fry girl he ever had! And the restaurant was only three blocks from my house, so I could easily walk back and forth to work.

The Sears and Roebuck store was close to our house, too. I took my sisters there to buy new clothes with my first paycheck. Kids always made fun of us for the clothes we wore to school, and I wanted them to have nicer ones so their schoolmates wouldn't pick on them anymore. I was excited for them and proud they would go to school in the clothes that I could buy for them.

I was ugly, poor, and essentially raising my siblings...

I bought myself a pair of white painter's pants with my next check. They were all the rage in the mid-seventies, and I couldn't wait to have a pair. The paycheck after that, I got contact lenses. As it turned out, though, it took more than white painter's pants and contact lenses for the other kids to stop tormenting me. The term used today is bullying. I was ugly, poor, and essentially raising my siblings: three strikes and you're out. These things made me a target and were not conducive to making friends. Different clothing and accessories could not change this situation. My persona, real or imagined, was already established.

But getting that fry job when I was fifteen began my foodservice career. For the first time in my life, I found a real sense of purpose and a sense of belonging. I made friends there, met my first serious boyfriend, and discovered my career path.

It's probably no surprise that I preferred work to school, though I did well in my studies. Looking back, I believe I was bored in school. Based on my previous statements, you can assume school was not my favorite place to be. This does not mean that I didn't do my work. I did. I am very fortunate that I tend to learn things quickly. I would always make sure I had my homework done and did well on exams.

But I didn't feel my physical presence was necessary (I am cringing as I write this—it sounds ridiculous). If I could work, I went to work instead of school. If one of my siblings were sick, I would have to stay home and care for them because my mom couldn't take off work. At least when I was home, no one was harassing me, and I wasn't the kid someone was forced to partner with because no one chose her.

All of this started in elementary school, and I remember crying and begging my mom not to make me go to school. I would cry the entire walk to school. Of course, none of my teachers knew what was happening in my home, or at school, for that matter. By the time I got to high school, I was over it, all of it: the bullying, life at home, everything. Work would be my way out of this unimaginable mess I was living. Of course, I had to get through high school first. Even though my work was always complete and my grades were good, a few teachers over the years thought my absenteeism was due to laziness or being indifferent. Rather than ask questions, they chose to demean me and become part of the problem rather than a potential solution. At least one teacher told me I'd never amount to anything. I wish he were still alive and I could find him. I'm sure he'd be surprised.

I stayed with that first foodservice corporation for more than twenty years, and I learned a lot. The world doesn't realize the skill sets you can develop and fine-tune over years working in foodservice (in any service industry, really). We learn people skills, analytical skills, communication skills, empathy, adaptability, self-control, patience, time management, and the list goes on.

That song "I'm Gonna Be Somebody" popped back in my head as I started my own company twenty-plus years, a second husband, and two children later. I couldn't have done it without the support of my family. My husband and my children are amazing. No matter what I accomplish, I will always tell you, without a doubt, being a mom and raising my children is the most important thing I've ever done.

So much happened between the time that fifteen-year-old girl started work at the fry station in a local fast-food restaurant and the time the nearly fifty-year-old woman started her own business. It's unfathomable to me that they are the same person, but they are.

This book is a snapshot of a few of those transformative years—the ones spent as a health inspector, attempting to protect my community's health while doing the best I could to educate the people who ran the food establishments I inspected. I've sprinkled this story with some food safety tidbits, too, and added a few personal life experiences that are sure to make you wonder how I survived my formative years.

TWO

Fry Girl at 15, Million-Dollar Budget at 24

I began my foodservice career at fifteen as a fry girl in a quick-service restaurant and left that establishment as an operating partner, more than twenty years later. I had many opportunities come my way during my time in operations, and I took advantage of as many as possible. The company offered educational reimbursement, training programs within the corporation itself, and years of diverse experience on the job. By the time I turned twenty-four, I was the general manager of a brand-spanking-new, million-dollar restaurant with more than seventy employees, and I was going to be the best damn manager they had ever seen!

My colleagues and I frequently discuss the myriad
skill sets this industry teaches.

I managed that location for more than fifteen years, and my team and I broke many sales records and won many awards. I loved my job. But running a foodservice operation of any type is far from easy. I'm frustrated to hear people talk down the industry, because I know how many skills I—and other foodservice workers—developed on the job. It taught me tolerance, patience, negotiation, people skills, how to handle volatile situations—and those are just the tip of the iceberg.

My colleagues and I frequently discuss the myriad skill sets this in-dustry teaches.

You can't imagine how angry people will sometimes get when they ask for a cheeseburger without pickles, and they inadvertently get one that has pickles on it. Or they get a Dr. Pepper when they asked for a Coke. One customer hurled his beverage back through the drive-thru window right at my cashier. He went home that day with reimburse-ment, but no food. I have never tolerated blatant acts of rudeness and disrespect.

In addition to people skills, I learned in that job how to handle a million-dollar budget, understand a profit and loss statement, address human resource issues, control payroll, and stay abreast of regulatory requirements. I made sales and budget projections. I managed marketing plans, food and cleaning supply costs, capital expenses, and repair and maintenance expenses while making a profit, and so...much...more. These are just some of the things the foodservice industry teaches us.

During the sixteen years I was at this facility, I managed thousands of employees. Many kids worked their way through high school and then college there. It was no easy feat to manage schedules around their extracurricular activities like football, soccer, baseball, band, and senior plays, not to mention family vacations. I prided myself on accommodating their needs, and as a result, I had one of the best teams in the company.

These kids and their families appreciated what I did for them and, in return, they were dedicated, hardworking, and loyal. Nothing made me more proud than when they earned significant accomplishments, whether it was an award, graduation, scholarships, or when the FBI, CIA, Defense Security Service, or any other branch appeared at my counter to perform a security clearance for a team member going into government work. Team members getting married, having babies, and welcoming new grandchildren were all momentous occasions we celebrated together.

All these years later, I'm still in touch with several of my employ-ees. When I started managing at that location, my own children were toddlers. When I left, my son was in high school, my daughter was in college, and they both were working there.

Time flies.

I was pretty removed from my peers in the industry, though, because my store was located in the country. At the time, women didn't hold positions of authority in this very rural area of the country. Many didn't make any important decisions on their own. I will never forget the first time I asked a young lady if she would work late, and she replied, "I have to call my husband to ask if I am allowed."

I was shocked. But I learned this was common. Most of the women called to get permission. Not to let their husband know they were working late—that I am totally on board with, as it's the respectful thing for either person in a relationship to do—but to get permission to work late.

It took quite a while for the community to adjust
to a woman being in a position of authority.

One day the fire chief came in and asked to speak to "the manager." I told him I was the manager. He said, "No, the real manager."

I laughed and said that I was the real manager.

He did not like that. He could see a supervisor in the back of the house. He pointed to him and said, "Go get that guy."

Whatever, I thought. "That guy" reported to me.

I yelled for the supervisor to come to the front. The fire chief asked him if we would donate cups to a fundraiser for an upcoming event. The supervisor looked at him, then at me, said, "You're going to have to ask her," and walked away.

The look on the fire chief's face was priceless. A female managing men, their children, handling customer service issues—it took quite a while for the community to adjust to a woman being in a position of authority. I liked to fondly compare it to Mayberry R.F.D. Still do.

As it turned out, I gained an unrealistic view of the "real world" at that job. I assumed everyone operated as I did. I am, by nature, an overachiever. My employees loathed this part of me, especially when I asked them to clean the drain covers, the wheels on the equipment, and the thresholds of the doors—with a toothbrush. I honestly thought all good managers had overnight cleaning parties, served pizza, and executed the extra cleaning activities alongside their employees. This is something I did regularly with my team. While we were working all night, scrubbing baseboards, cleaning vents, deep cleaning urinals and floor drains, we had fun—as crazy as it sounds. It wasn't our typical day. There was music, pizza, conversation, and I was there cleaning with them. It helped build morale, respect, and commitment.

Most managers didn't even own a flashlight, let alone use one to look under the equipment to see if it was clean.

One of my daughter's friends still talks about her first night working there. Apparently, I made her clean the grout in the wall behind the chicken station (I'm sure she used a toothbrush—there was no shortage of them, and they do the job so well). I don't remember, but she does—some twenty years later. I must have made quite an impression.

Later on life's journey, I found out I was terribly wrong. Not everyone took this cleaning and sanitation thing nearly as seriously as I did. Most managers didn't even own a flashlight, let alone use one to look under the equipment to see if it was clean.

All of my major life milestones happened while I worked for this company. I turned sixteen, learned how to drive, started dating, turned eighteen, graduated from high school, got married, had my babies, bought my first house, lost my mom, and the list goes on. The company was as much a part of me as my heart was.

In 2003, for various reasons, it was time to leave this company that I had loved for more than half of my life. I thought my career in foodservice was over. But it was only the beginning.

THREE

My First Day

W hen I began conducting food safety inspections, I was so excited —and more naive than I am pleased to admit.

When I first left the fast-food restaurant, I developed and ran educational programs for many corporations, explaining how important a good food safety culture is. So by this point in my career, I had educated several thousand people in food safety, from hourly employees to senior executives at independent restaurants and large corporations. I had worked as a national trainer and third-party inspector for a few years. I had started my own company, Food Safety Training Solutions, LLC, in 2008, which had rebranded to Savvy Food Safety a few years later.

Savvy Food Safety has since been contracted for many things, including third-party inspections, regulatory inspections, academic classes, and private sector contracts. I've spoken around the world, hosted podcasts, and founded two other companies.

But back when I first started food safety inspections under my own company's name, I was fresh and enthusiastic from the success of my educational programs. I was sure I would 100 percent enjoy this new journey on which I was about to embark. After all, everyone wants to get a good score on their health inspection, right?

On my first day as an inspector, I was filled with ambition, as I always am, anticipating that foodservice operations would welcome their new health inspector. I assumed everyone wanted to make a good first impression. If there's one person you don't want to piss off in the restaurant biz, it's your health inspector, right? That's what they always told me, and I believed it to be true. Apparently not.

I jumped in the car with my assistant to begin my day. I donned my freshly pressed white lab coat, new ID, and an appropriate hat. I double-checked to be sure I had all the proper tools with me: a brand new, calibrated thermometer for accurate temperature taking; a flashlight for peeking under equipment, up grill hoods, and in hidden nooks and crannies; a UV light to look for evidence of rodents; sanitizer testing strips; and a camera to take pictures as evidence.

We had a forty-minute drive to our first stop, plenty of time to chat about the locations we would visit, the order of visits, how we'd approach the people in charge (PICs), and what my assistant's role would be as we moved through the day.

We parked the car, gathered our items, and headed for the first establishment. I opened the door to the small restaurant with a smile on my face and an extended hand to introduce myself, anticipating a cordial response at a minimum.

Imagine my surprise when the manager's response to my arrival was, "Health inspector? You're going to have to schedule an appointment!"

"Excuse me?" I replied.

"You heard me. You're going to have to schedule an appointment!" she snapped.

"I'm sorry, that's not how this works."

"Well, the old inspector always called ahead," she responded.

"When was your last inspection?" I asked.

She retorted, "Four years ago!" I didn't believe her, but I played along.

"Wow, I guess you are surprised to see me. I won't be scheduling my visits. They will be unannounced, and I will stop by to say hi twice a year." I said it with a smile through clenched teeth, working my way to the back of the facility. And that is how my journey began—not quite as I had hoped.

I moved on to my next facility, and someone with a similar demeanor met me at the counter.

"Ma'am, we don't get inspected," the manager said sternly.

I replied, "You're on my list. I will do your inspection today."

"You can't! I need to get ready. I will call when you can come back!" he snarled.

"When was your last inspection?" I asked.

"Four years. It's been at least four years. I told you we don't get inspected!"

"Beginning today, I will do an inspection twice a year," I said.

Let's just say health inspections are so different when you have an inspector who takes her job seriously. My first week was brutal! Other PICs met me with similar comments:

"I haven't been inspected in four years!"

"I don't get inspected!"

"You need to schedule an appointment!"

"The inspector just drops by, and I sign a form!"

What?

I was the only health inspector in this town, and currently, the consensus was that I was stirring up trouble.

I came to realize the PICs were telling me the truth. Most of them had not seen a health inspector in a very long time. What in the world had I walked into? One thing was for sure, reining in the situation would be difficult, very difficult. I was the only health inspector in this town, and currently, the consensus was that I was stirring up trouble.

"You won't last long."

I heard those words multiple times during my first month. I took it as a challenge. Who dares to tell the health inspector they "won't last long"? Maybe they mistook my diminutive stature for vulnerability. *Big* mistake.

Each facility was on my schedule to inspect twice a year. Once during the first half of the year and again in the second half of the year, in no specific order—and trust me, I did them randomly. I came from operations. I knew what they'd expect. There was no chance I would walk out of one restaurant in a strip mall and walk into the restaurant next door. Nor would I inspect one location of a brand, then immediately head to another branch of that same brand elsewhere in town. Are you kidding me? When the health inspector is in the area, phones are ringing off the hook throughout the entire town. Other locations of each brand you walk into are warned, so they can "get ready." No. My schedule was random. Problem solved.

Years before I became a health inspector, I conducted third-party inspections for several large casinos, and we went through several phases. When I began doing the inspections, the brand managers and executive chefs didn't know my name, but as soon as I inspected the first restaurant, every facility in the casino knew I was in the house.

If a facility knows when an inspector will show up,
they'll prepare for the inspection.

These inspections were always unannounced, even though they were third party. Inspectors should handle all third-party reviews this way. Otherwise, they lack integrity. If a facility knows when an inspector will show up, they'll prepare for the inspection. When the auditor or inspector walks in the door, they get an inaccurate picture of reality.

Eventually they realized I showed up once a quarter, so the chefs called the front desk and asked the hotel manager to let them know when I made reservations—crafty little devils. I caught on when there was a sudden spike in everyone's inspection score. So, feeling like a celebrity, and with the assistance of the VP of Food and Beverage, I began checking in under aliases. Problem solved.

Now, I tend to be a creature of habit, and I would order room service while I settled into my room and changed for the inspection. Common sense said I couldn't go to any of the restaurants to eat. I realized the room service personnel would recognize me, but you can only do so much to prepare for an inspection in thirty minutes.

I never gave a thought to my order. These trips were long. I would inspect three or four casinos at a time, and each of them might have as many as ten kitchens and restaurants—maybe more. Energy drinks were my savior. Mmmm, but who else was ordering energy drinks from room service at 6:00 a.m.? It turns out they kept them on hand in the room service area just for *me*! OMG. *Busted.* I had to laugh.

Even still, it was maybe forty-five minutes notice from the time I placed my order for an energy drink until I walked into the first kitchen. There is not a lot of work you can do in that amount of time in those kitchens to hide noncompliance, especially when they are busy. After I made that discovery, I stopped ordering room service. My husband regularly hid snacks in my suitcase, and I learned to call them breakfast.

FOUR

The Emergency Calls and Special Events

People often ask, "What is the most bizarre experience you ever had when working in a restaurant?"

I always need clarification on that question, because I'm confident they don't intend to speak with me for the next several hours. We can talk about when I worked in foodservice or when I conducted health inspections. Those are two very different scenarios. Each can be equally disturbing.

I've already told you some of the bizarre situations throughout my career in both roles, but there were many, many more.

Everyone at the front counter disappeared and left the pregnant girl there alone.

When one transfers to a new facility, there's always a bit of a learning curve. It takes a bit to get acclimated to the new atmosphere. Good or not, it's an adjustment, as change is with any job. And if you are in a position of authority, especially if you are very young—I was twenty-one—the employees will "test" you.

One evening as we were preparing to close, an employee walked up to me and said, "There's a fish in the toilet!"

"Ummmm, excuse me?"

I thought he was joking. Why would there be a goldfish in the toilet at a restaurant? I said as much to him.

His response: "I didn't say it was a goldfish. It's a trout."

What the hell? Sure enough, there was a slimy dead trout in the toilet of the men's room. *I wonder how long they intend to keep me in this restaurant*, I thought.

Another time, when I was pregnant with my daughter, a gentleman came in, ordered a roast beef sandwich, and stood at the counter talking about the FBI surveilling him and warning that we'd better not poison his sandwich. Everyone at the front counter disappeared and left the pregnant girl there alone.

I was alone at the front counter with a furious man who thought the FBI was following him and trying to kill him.

Though it only took a minute or two to get his meal together, the longer he stood waiting at the counter, the more enraged he became! I handed him his bag, and out the door he went. Phew, we were happy that was over. My coworkers began to reappear one by one, and—*holy crap*—here he came back in the door with his unopened bag of food.

Once again, I was alone at the front counter with a furious man who thought the FBI was following him and trying to kill him.

We didn't have security systems in those days, no alarms under the front counter, no cell phones. I prayed I would not give birth then and there and hoped one of my employees had the foresight to dial 911 before this man pulled me over the counter.

He began ripping the bag and screaming at me about the FBI, which now included alien involvement. He was literally shredding the food as he tore at the bag. Food flew *everywhere*—French fries, shreds of roast beef, and pieces of bun. I had food in my hair.

If it hadn't been so sad, it would have been funny.

All this was witnessed by an older woman who came in late every afternoon and liked to sit in the first booth until late in the evening. This booth was in direct view of the front counter.

Now, it's best to brace yourself for what I am about to tell you. If you have a weak stomach, skip a paragraph or two.

Every day she came in, ordered a cup of coffee, sat in that same booth for hours, and picked her nose, rolling the remnants into a ball. That's right, every day. She'd put the booger ball in her pocket for safekeeping overnight and bring it out again as she sat down. It grew bigger every day. The unhinged man at the front counter had this poor woman so flustered on this particular day that she threw the booger ball. And that upset her, because she had lost her prized possession.

As the police arrived, the woman was frantically searching for her trophy while we tried to reassure the gentleman at the front counter that the FBI was not present, and the aliens had gone home. Thank God for the men in blue. (I say men because they were men.)

After I started working with the health department, I received a phone call from the secretary telling me that someone filed a complaint saying they found a cockroach in their bowl of soup. Any time there's a complaint, an inspector must follow up on it within a specific timeframe. So the following day, I scheduled that restaurant as my first stop. Unless there is a significant infestation, cockroaches don't typically end up in random bowls of soup.

As an inspector, I know where to look for cockroaches, and it doesn't take long to find them if there really is an infestation. I walked into the kitchen and began removing panels from the refrigeration equipment. Cockroaches love warm, moist, dark places. As soon as I took the first panel off a food prep case, cockroaches scattered. There were so many, you couldn't even see the metal fins on the condenser, but they started to run as soon as the light hit them. The facility definitely needed a visit from a pest control operator (PCO) and to be put on a regular maintenance program.

Most of the time, vendors that show up for special events are prepared for a visit from the health inspector, knowing they need an inspection in order to get their permit for the event. They receive all of this information when they submit their application to serve at the event, and they are not allowed to operate without that permit.

Still, some vendors would arrive without handwashing facilities, hand soap, or single-use gloves. Sometimes they wouldn't have any way to wash their dishes. If an operator doesn't care enough to make sure their facility has the basics to function safely, how could I, in good conscience, permit them to sell food to the public? I couldn't. So they didn't, regardless of how far they drove to get there or how upset they were.

Many times I heard the same story I had been hearing for months—they'd been coming here for years and no one had inspected them, or inspectors had just signed their forms. Sometimes I felt really bad about the situation, but I assure you I would have felt much worse if someone got sick or died on my watch.

During my tenure, vendors never showed up to an event unprepared more than once. The next time they came to our community, they brought everything they needed to operate safely. They knew they wouldn't be permitted to sell any of their temperature-controlled products if they didn't. The risk to the general public was too significant for me to allow them that privilege if they couldn't follow the guidelines they knew were a requirement.

I needed a new thermometer and a few other items one day, so I stopped in at the local restaurant supply store. Many of the restaurants were not using thermometers and didn't have them in their kitchens. It was the same situation with sanitizer test strips. I'd dropped my thermometer and needed a new one, and I was out of test strips. I couldn't find the test strips on the sales floor of the supply shop, so I asked the clerk if they had any in the stockroom.

She evidently didn't realize who I was, because she launched into a tirade about what a bitch the new health inspector must be. She said her shop was selling out of everything. They didn't have any sanitizer test strips or sanitizer buckets, they were nearly out of thermometers, and on and on. I let her talk as she wrote up my order. When she was finished, I asked her for an invoice.

She said, "Sure, hon, what's your name?"

I replied very calmly, "Francine. I'm the health inspector." I took the invoice out of her hand, turned around, and walked out the door.

The expression on her face was priceless.

Some would think the shop might be grateful for the increase in sales. After all, they were the only restaurant supply store in town. The salesclerk was likely frustrated managing stock levels, so she regurgitated information to explain why she was currently out of so many items. It wasn't her fault; it was the new bitch of a health inspector's.

I had discovered many years prior that you learn more if you keep your mouth shut and let people talk. My getting defensive would have served no purpose. I was well aware that individuals purchasing supplies from her were not happy with me.

As I got into my car to drive away, I smiled to myself. I wondered if the past few minutes had taught her anything about customer service and being careful what she said to others in general. I hoped for the best.

FIVE

Norovirus: It's Common and It's Ugly

Every year there are numerous, widespread, severe foodborne illness outbreaks. Many in the foodservice industry think it won't happen to them. But it can happen to anyone at any time, and it does.

The Chipotle enterprise prides itself on "food with integrity," but the restaurant chain had multiple reports of foodborne illness outbreaks between 2015 and 2018. These outbreaks ultimately cost them over twenty-five million dollars to resolve criminal charges related to the incidents.

They also cost the company millions of dollars in litigation costs, settlements, plummeting stocks, and lost sales. Not to mention, it takes significant time, money, and energy to rebuild the brand after that kind of negative fallout. Some organizations—like ChiChis—never recover from a foodborne illness outbreak. They simply go out of business.

Many of Chipotle's outbreaks involved norovirus. It seemed like every news article I was asked to write during that time involved Chipotle. I eventually had to say no. I worried that it looked like I had a personal vendetta against the brand. I didn't.

Chipotle was repeatedly mentioned in the media as an example of what not to do, but they have also been cited as an excellent case study on how to recover from such tragedies. Which is no easy task.

Once the public's trust is lost, it's tough to regain. Most never manage it. In Chipotle's case, society seems to have forgiven them, and they seem willing to learn from their mistakes. The company also took responsibility for their errors. That doesn't make the errors okay, but it sure beats denials, lying, and kicking and screaming the entire way through the judicial system, as some other companies have done.

In 2014, the exclusive Mohonk Mountain House resort, located in New Paltz, NY, had a norovirus outbreak that made hundreds of visitors ill and nearly shut down the Valentine's Day tourism sales. This outbreak culminated in a class action lawsuit.

All of these companies have corporate policies and procedures to protect against foodborne illness, yet something still went wrong. The risk is real for every company serving food.

I assure you, there are things on that doorknob you do not want on your freshly cleaned hands.

As a customer, there are a few things you can do to protect yourself.

Wash your hands with soap and warm water. Use a paper towel to grasp the water faucet—you don't want anyone else's poop on your hands, and everyone has turned on the water! If paper towels are available, use them to dry your hands rather than an air dryer. The clean paper towel helps to remove any additional germs you may have missed. Use a paper towel to open the door. I assure you, there are things on that doorknob you do not want on your freshly cleaned hands. Norovirus is only one of them (as of the writing of this book, that includes the COVID variants).

Warm-air hand dryers sometimes use fan speeds of over 370 miles per hour, strong enough to spread pathogens in the air as far as 5 feet from the drying unit. In addition, pathogens can be scattered onto your clothing, increasing the spread of those contaminants. Those pathogens can also linger in the air for up to 15 minutes.

One of the main complaints about paper towels is the problem of waste—they're not part of the sustainable ecosystem. However, paper towels are now designed so we can compost them after use. That puts them back into the system. Additionally, paper towels can be sustainably sourced, or made from recycled materials, to minimize the environmental effects.

Typical norovirus symptoms include projectile vomiting, explosive diarrhea, nausea, and stomach pain. You may also experience fever, headache, and body aches. Many think this is the flu. It is not.

The flu is a respiratory infection. The cause of *this* hideous illness is eating contaminated food, drinking contaminated water, or touching your hand to your mouth after it has been in contact with a contaminated surface or item. These items have an invisible smudge of infected feces, and it can take as few as ten norovirus particles to cause illness. Think faucet, doorknob, gas pump, stylus or keypad at the checkout, elevator button, remote control, or any of the dozens of other things you randomly touch every day.

Norovirus is the number one foodborne illness in the world, with an estimated 685 million cases per year globally. Nearly 200 million of these cases are children under 5 years old, leading to about 50,000 needless deaths of children a year.

I entered the restroom to wash my hands
and noticed there was no hot water.

In the United States, 58 percent of foodborne illness outbreaks are norovirus, the equivalent of about 2,500 reported annual outbreaks. This foodborne illness causes about 900 deaths, about 465,000 emergency room visits, and 19–21 million illnesses annually. This is 100 percent preventable. *All* foodborne illnesses are preventable.

I entered a popular hot spot one day to do a health inspection during the late lunch hour. I entered the restroom to wash my hands and noticed there was no hot water. Odd, as the restroom was directly on the opposite side of the kitchen wall.

I walked to the front counter, made the appropriate introductions, and wandered into the kitchen. I went directly to the utility room, which housed the water heater, and found it turned off. Not broken, not a pilot out, but turned off.

If the water heater was off, it meant there was no hot water in the building. Customers filled the dining room, and an employee was hand-washing dishes. They did not have a mechanical dishwasher, and no one seemed to be aware there was a problem. These are all things I observed very quickly, in just a few seconds.

It's how health inspectors' minds are trained to work—all while thinking about the potential risks involved. Often employees are innocently our best resource, so I asked one about the hot water situation. He told me the manager turned it off all the time to save money. Well, that explained why everything else seemed to be operating status quo and no one appeared concerned about the lack of hot water, including for the dishwasher!

The water may have been cold, but my blood was boiling. It didn't take me long to find the manager.

I had no possible way to know which dishes had been adequately washed, rinsed, and sanitized. Or how long or how often the manager had been implementing this "money-saving" procedure. There was only one way to correct a problem like this. Close the restaurant and make them wash every single dish, glass, and utensil in the place. So that is what I did.

How much money did the manager think he was saving, and at whose expense? The hot water was only one of many issues at that location. It was one of those days when I truly worried they might lock me in the freezer. Fortunately, they didn't.

Let me give you a quick tip: in most cases, foodservice facilities only have one water heater. If you let the hot water run in the restroom for a while and it doesn't produce any hot water, they likely don't have any in the kitchen, either.

Go someplace else to eat.

There are a few exceptions—extensive facilities such as casinos have multiple kitchens and multiple resources. But your smaller, stand-alone restaurants are the ones to note. No hot water in the restroom should make you question whether there's hot water in the kitchen.

SIX

A Shout-Out to Fast Food!

Did you know the number one restaurant in the world had a foodborne illness outbreak?

I want to give a shout-out to fast-food restaurants. These places take a beating in the media and from the public. But a foodborne illness outbreak can happen in any kind of food establishment—fast, casual, fine dining, potluck, or in your own home! Yes, your own home. Your kitchen is more disgusting than you know.

Noma was voted The World's Best Restaurant three years in a row by The World's 50 Best Restaurants list before having a norovirus outbreak in 2013. This restaurant was charging up to $260 ($339 adjusted for inflation in 2023, the time of publication) for a menu without drinks, and reservations often had to be made months in advance.

America's food industry has a $55.5 billion food safety problem, including foodborne illness outbreaks. (Remember, an outbreak occurs when two or more people get the same illness from the same contaminated food or drink.) The list below represents some of the 2021 and 2022 investigations in which the CDC was the lead public health agency for multistate foodborne outbreaks. Keep in mind that all foodborne illnesses are preventable. In many of the outbreaks listed below, people died needlessly.

- Packaged Salads: *E. coli* O157:H7

- Fresh Express Packaged Salads: *Listeria monocytogenes*
- Dole Packaged Salads: *Listeria monocytogenes*
- Baby Spinach: *E. coli* O157:H7
- Salami Sticks: *Salmonella* I 4,[5],12:i:-
- Seafood: *Salmonella* Thompson
- Onions: *Salmonella* Oranienburg
- Italian-Style Meats: *Salmonella* infections
- Cake Mix: *E. coli* O121
- Prepackaged Salads: *Salmonella* Typhimurium
- Fully Cooked Chicken: *Listeria monocytogenes*
- Frozen Cooked Shrimp: *Salmonella* Weltevreden
- Raw Frozen Breaded Stuffed Chicken Products: *Salmonella* Enteritidis
- Cashew Brie: *Salmonella* Duisburg
- Ground Turkey: *Salmonella* Hadar
- Queso Fresco: *Listeria monocytogenes*
- Unknown Food Source: *E. coli* O157:H7

As I write this, we are only a few days into 2023, and already *three* people have died because they ate at a restaurant and contracted hepatitis A. And there will likely be more deaths. Wash your freaking hands, people. There is no excuse.

Everyone who works in the foodservice industry should be concerned about sickening or even killing customers with a foodborne illness. That means everyone from the farmers that grow the food to the restaurants that serve it should take every precaution to reduce that risk. While the main concern is keeping consumers safe, it's also important to realize that *foodborne illnesses can be costly and damaging for businesses.*

A foodborne illness incident or outbreak can cost foodservice professionals (farmers, restaurants, hotels, manufacturers, retailers, etc.) significant money through decreased revenues, high legal fees, potential lawsuits, and diminished sales and loyalty from concerned customers. A severely damaged reputation could permanently shut a company's doors. Remember that $55.5 billion is the annual cost of foodborne illnesses in medical treatment, lost productivity, and illness-related mortality in the United States.

According to a study from researchers at Johns Hopkins Bloomberg School of Public Health, the cost of a *single foodborne illness outbreak* at a fast-food restaurant could be between $3,968 and $1.9 million, depending on the severity of the epidemic; the number of lawsuits, fines, and legal fees; and the number of people impacted by the incident. And the costs for other kinds of establishments are even higher. According to the study, costs per incident are $6,330 to $2.1 million for fast-casual establishments; $8,030 to $2.2 million for casual dining restaurants; and $8,273 to $2.6 million for fine dining restaurants.

It doesn't matter if we discuss fine dining, quick service, fast food, or food trucks. There are high quality and low quality in all of them, and I've seen it all.

I've inspected fast-food restaurants where you could damn near eat off the floor.

I've been in fine dining restaurants storing marinara sauce and "mystery meat" in old chemical buckets kept on the floor of filthy walk-in coolers (and, of course, the products didn't have labels or dates). Conversely, I've inspected fast-food restaurants where you could damn near eat off the floor. It's unfortunate that it's always these establishments that get beaten up all the time about the quality of their stores and the food they serve. When I hear those insidious comments, I am the first to stop the perpetrator in their tracks. It's all about the operator running the restaurant.

When you work in my field, you can walk into a restaurant and know the manager's strengths within the first few minutes. Most possess a more robust skill set in one area than another. One operator's strengths might be cleaning and maintenance, and another manager might focus on customer service, marketing, and running their business profitably. The goal should be to assemble a complementary management staff— where one member is weak, another is strong. If everyone is focused on cleaning, the unit will be spotless but customer service might be terrible. Now and then, a rare, well-rounded gem is strong in multiple skill sets.

I can think of one restaurant chain that is consistently on top of things everywhere I go. That's it—just one chain. And by consistent, I'm going to say the quality is maintained at 98 percent of locations I visit across the country. I always wonder: If they can do it, why can't everyone? It is by no means an easy task, but apparently it can be done.

I had a Chinese restaurant in my jurisdiction that was always meticulous. The facility was clean and organized, the products were all properly labeled with names and dates, and personal hygiene standards were on point. The entire time I was their health inspector, I never had an issue.

And I love Chinese food, so occasionally that spot would be my restaurant of choice for dinner when I was done with work for the day. The gentleman who owned the restaurant was beside himself with excitement whenever I ate there. He would greet me in the parking lot, open the door for me, and attempt to give me special dishware and Western utensils. It was a sweet gesture. But while I appreciated his efforts, and I didn't want to offend him, it was inappropriate for me to allow this to happen.

I could not allow the perception that I was provided any special favors by anyone at any facility.

Each time, I made him take away the table settings and serve my food in standard dishes, with chopsticks. Half the fun of eating Chinese for me is eating with chopsticks. I could not allow the perception that I was provided any special favors by anyone at any facility. Allowing the table settings would undoubtedly create that perception. But there's no more profound compliment to a restaurant than for the health inspector to eat at their facility, and this gentleman was over the moon every time I stepped in the door.

As health inspectors, we must know how our actions impact our jobs. I never ate or drank anything at any of the facilities when I was working, and I never accepted anything offered to me, not even water, as it could be perceived as a bribe. Honesty and integrity are fundamental to me and critical to doing the job, and I did my best to remain above reproach.

There is both exceptional and poor quality in all foodservice establishments, to some degree, whether you pay two dollars for a cheeseburger or ninety-nine dollars for a three-course meal.

We can go back to the example of Noma, the establishment in Copenhagen, Denmark that was the number one restaurant in the world for some time. Noma's kitchen is known for being pristine, and it is undoubtedly high dollar. But a high-dollar restaurant doesn't guarantee the kitchen is pristine. And clean doesn't guarantee you won't get sick. In 2013, Noma sickened sixty-seven individuals with norovirus—the number one foodborne illness globally.

I understand that bad experiences happen, but the positives certainly outweigh the negatives.

Negative comments about people who work in the foodservice industry are common, especially in fast food. They are consistently referred to as burger flippers, stupid, lazy, and worse. Most of these individuals are anything but lazy and stupid, and they certainly do more than flip burgers. I understand that bad experiences happen, but the positives certainly outweigh the negatives. We simply hear about the negatives more often.

Social media has enabled negative reviews to travel the world in seconds, true or not. And customers who have a terrible experience are two to three times more likely to post comments and write a negative review than those who have a great experience are to write a positive review. It takes about twelve positive comments to cancel out the nasty effects of one bad review.

Humans spend more time analyzing and picking apart bad experiences than thinking about positive encounters, too, which is an annoying fact of human nature. And unfortunately, for too many, perception is reality. I am afraid there isn't much that will change the perception of fast-food employees anytime soon. But I will tell you that it takes an upbeat and open personality, patience, and a solid sense of humor to work in fast food.

Along with those traits, one must be able to multitask, follow verbal and written instructions, and work as part of a team while demonstrating manual dexterity, physical stamina, and the ability to diffuse angry customers—all under pressure.

These do not sound like traits of stupid, lazy people. I will tell you, some of the people I've encountered in the industry are the most brilliant and hardest working people I know. I'm proud to call them my friends.

In the end, most businesses try to do the right thing, but there are anomalies, and I believe they are unfortunately more common than we think. Please don't assume it's only fast-food restaurants that will make you sick. I'll talk about your own kitchen at home later. It's filthier than you think!

SEVEN

I Never Wanted to Be "That" Person

When I worked in corporate America, we would occasionally have VIP visits from senior executives. As the general manager of a restaurant that performed very well, I always seemed to end up on their visit list. Since then, I've realized that no one else scrubbed their drains or the grout in their floors with a toothbrush. Silly me.

These visits were always such a dog and pony show, but being the overachiever I am—and never one to disappoint—I'd strive to exceed expectations. Looking to achieve a level of perfection that is not (really!) attainable, I'd go to great lengths to make my superiors look good, too. Many times for not so much as a thank you.

On one such occasion, the company chose my restaurant as one of the units the company president would visit. Keep in mind, the next store in the chain nearest to mine was some thirty miles away. I was very rural—in the middle of nowhere. This visit by the president was a *big* deal!

And every executive at every level of management between myself and him got on my every last nerve by nagging me in the run-up to the visit. I would make sure nothing went wrong. If they needed to be that concerned, why was he visiting my store?

Before the visit, I decided the surface of my concrete sidewalks should be whiter than the day they were poured. So I went to the hardware store and bought some muriatic acid. I spent a fair amount of time outside cleaning my sidewalks the morning of the company president's arrival.

I never gave any thought to the worms in the ground alongside the sidewalk. I just knew that time was running out, the president would be there soon, and I had to hurry up and wash those sidewalks! I nearly fainted when I realized the acid hurt the worms. I didn't intend to kill them! Nor did I want a bunch of dead worms lying around on top of my mulch right outside the door he'd have to walk through when he showed up!

And here I was, shuffling around with the soles flapping off
the bottom of my shoes.

When I was finished scrubbing the walk and putting everything away, I realized the acid had eaten the threads out of my new shoes. The soles were falling off! This man would show up in a matter of hours, and I'd be running around in a new, freshly pressed uniform, in a store that was so clean you could eat off the bathroom floor or the sidewalk (well, almost)—and my shoes were soleless.

Now, what the hell would I do?! I am sure you're thinking: go to the store to get a pair, duh. I did mention the restaurant was in a rural area. Very rural. So it wasn't that easy. The nearest place to buy a pair of shoes was nearly an hour one way away, even if I didn't obey the speed limit. No time for that.

I had even cleaned my restaurant's hose, the hose we used to hot-hose the floors throughout the building at night. That thing must have been seventy-five feet long, and when I say clean, I mean we scrubbed and waxed that pink rubber hose so it looked brand new. And here I was, shuffling around with the soles flapping off the bottom of my shoes. Sweet Jesus. I was about to die.

My staff and I had put hours and hours of back-breaking work into this VIP visit. A tour of this magnitude occurred maybe twice during my entire career with this company. The pressure put on me by executive management to perform at the highest level, not to mention the pressure I put on myself, was excessive. But we did it. Not one negative comment, not even about my soleless shuffle. (I had deliberately stayed out of the way as much as possible during the day.)

Mission accomplished. Thank you, team. Without them, who was I?

Because my workers always rose to the challenges I gave them, I always took care of my staff. There is never a need, as owners and managers in foodservice, or any other business, to mistreat your staff. The same is true for customers. The general public doesn't have the right to mistreat service personnel, either. There's nothing a staff member can do that would give you the right to verbally or physically abuse them. Nothing.

I know everyone has a bad day now and then, and people can get a little irritated. Okay, I can deal with that. But when the public starts calling my employees names, yelling at them, or throwing things at them, I will not tolerate that on any day.

If missing out on fries in your order or getting a Dr. Pepper instead of a Coke is the worst thing that happens in your day, your day has not been all that bad. It doesn't give you a reason to throw stuff at another human being.

On one crazy Friday night, we'd been slammed for hours. Suddenly, I saw a thirty-two-ounce beverage fly through the drive-thru window straight at one of my cashiers. What in the world? She was more than a little startled—obviously! I went to the window to see what happened and found out my cashier had inadvertently handed a customer the wrong beverage.

So, I get it—he wanted a different drink. But if he thought it was okay to throw his beverage at the seventeen-year-old girl working the window, he was sorely mistaken. I gave him his money back. And told him he could take his family somewhere else for dinner. They probably had to go home and cook. We were the only fast-food restaurant in town.

Another time a customer came to the front counter during a jam-packed evening and began berating a cashier who was busting her butt to take care of customers. He was mad because he was missing an order of fries. If he had given her a minute and told her his fries were missing, the cashier would have gone and gotten them for him—no questions. Instead, he walked up to the counter and began yelling and calling her names.

I remember asking him if I could help him. I told him the cashier didn't get paid enough to listen to him, but if he talked to me like that, he'd leave without the fries. I thought he'd pull me over the counter and strangle me. Fortunately that did not happen. I stood my ground as the cashier got the gentleman an order of fresh fries. She handed him his bag, thanked him, and he was on his way.

Oh, the stories. The craziness. The mistreatment. All so unnecessary. Most people have no idea.

A gentleman would come in late and enter the restroom almost every evening during what we called "pre-closing"—when everything in the dining room and restrooms has been cleaned and restocked. He was a retired doctor, and he always carried a can of Lysol. But after he left, there would be poop smeared all over the restroom wall.

I realized, OMG, I have become "that person," the regular.

Our customers weren't all bad. We had many regulars we loved. A few months ago, I stopped in at a convenience store on my way to the office, and instead of the girl I was used to seeing, a different girl waited on me. Suddenly I heard a voice behind her say, "She likes one kept out of the bag. Put the other two inside. She'll be back in a few days. She always gets the same order." And then my regular cashier looked at me and smiled. She was right.

It struck me as oddly comforting but discomforting at the same time. I realized, OMG, I have become "that person," the regular. The one who comes in predictably and gets the same thing with the same routine every time. I don't know why, but I felt suddenly anxious. I never wanted to be "that" person. I had an instant flashback to the predictable elderly folks who showed up at the same time every day, ordered the same meal consistently, and sat in the same seats. If anyone was in "their" seats, they would get upset—even angry—as if they owned that portion of the restaurant. And suddenly, I felt like one of them.

I spent more than two decades in operations and experienced customers with a broad range of personalities. Some became like family, some I watched grow old, and once I had to call a customer's family member when I was worried that dementia had set in for the customer, they were having a bad day, and maybe they shouldn't be driving. I attended funerals and surprise birthday parties for members of the "coffee club." Once, the gentleman who was fluent in Russian made me a sign in Russian for some Russian guests who were visiting our town. Those are great memories that can't be overshadowed by any outrageousness that occurred. Kids intentionally set a car on fire in our parking lot. The sink was ripped off our bathroom wall over and over again by couples feeling the need to have sex in the restroom. These were the kind of things that helped build character, gave me problem-solving skills, and taught me how to deal with adversity. While they weren't my best days at work, I certainly did learn from them and wouldn't change anything. They made me who I am today—and I have a tolerance level that most can't imagine.

EIGHT

One of My Favorite Restaurants—Not!

One of my favorite restaurants was in my jurisdiction for inspection. I was excited at a chance to meet the owners and see the back of the house, which I was sure would be as excellent as the marble floors in the lobby and the spectacular entrance into the building.

This facility is a fine dining establishment. They serve the most fantastic food, and it's considered a bit pricey. Many of their patrons only visit on special occasions—birthdays, anniversaries, and other celebratory events.

The mouth-watering crab au gratin and cream of crab soup here are to die for, the prime rib will make your taste buds dance, and the freshly created salads are served with a *chilled* fork! I'm talking about a place where kids go for prom dates, proposals happen, and wedding receptions are booked many months in advance. People make business deals here, judges and politicians take people for dinner, and the local doctors and lawyers have lunch. Corporations hold Christmas parties, schools have proms, and I have attended dozens of events here over the years.

My assistant and I entered the building through an elegantly hand-carved front door. It was early, a bit before lunch, and the hostess greeted us. I showed her my ID and asked to see the owner. I was anxious to meet him and get started.

A few minutes passed, and the owner eventually appeared in the lobby to greet me. I explained who I was, and she very hesitantly took me back to the kitchen. I quickly learned the establishment was not nearly as excited about my visit as I was! The owner's husband and co-owner began speaking to her, loudly and rapidly, in their native language. I don't know what he said, but it wasn't pleasant. She quickly left the kitchen. As their conversation was transpiring, I'd begun doing my thing.

I was instantly shell-shocked by what I saw in that kitchen.

Several shelving units lined the wall. They were about eight feet high and must have been four or five feet deep. The establishment had covered every shelf from floor to ceiling with sheets of quarter-inch plywood. The plywood was there to keep items from falling through the spaces in the shelving, but it was extremely dirty. Using the plywood this way was already a significant health code violation.

Who knows what he walked through before his shoes came in contact with those dishes.

But to make matters worse, an employee was on the third shelf from the bottom, crawling through the dishware on his hands and knees. I don't know what he was searching for, but all I could see was the bottom of his feet! Are you kidding me? The soles of his shoes were scraping across plates, saucers, cups, and multiple other food-contact surfaces. Who knows what he walked through before his shoes came in contact with those dishes. Dishes that guests would be eating lobster, crab, and filet mignon off of later that evening—with no knowledge that someone's feet had been all over them earlier in the day. They may have even seen him in the restroom, wearing those same shoes. Of course, I made the staff take every dish off those shelves and wash, rinse, and sanitize them before they could use them. They also had to rid the building of the plywood.

General filth was everywhere here, but the entire facility I walked through up front to get to this point was pristine!

Did I mention those chilled forks?

They were chilling on about an inch of filthy frost—quite literally dark gray. I wanted to cry. Having spent so many years in the industry myself, I am not unfamiliar with the difference between "working dirt" and "filth." What I saw was filth.

Upon entering the walk-in cooler, I observed several five-gallon chemical buckets. One was filled with marinara sauce, another with soup, and another with "mystery meat" and various animal bones—to this very day I honestly do not know what the hell was in that bucket. But I know they used whatever was in it to make their "amazing" soup.

I am rarely at a loss for words, but I had such a mix of emotions in that moment, it was difficult to control my fury. I was angry for five main reasons:

- This establishment was beyond disgusting in terms of filth.
- The price of the average plate was irrelevant, but their guests ate there thinking that they were getting something "special." They were paying a small fortune for a plate of food that could have very well made them sick, or even killed them. Much of the clientele was older, as younger people couldn't typically afford to eat there except for special occasions. It was memorable, all right.
- There were multiple "critical" food code violations, and it was clear the facility had been operating in this manner for a very long time.
- Cockroaches ran amok in the daylight. Workers would smash them and swipe them onto the floor like they were bread crumbs. Cockroaches can carry *Salmonella* and more, but there was no effort to even wipe the counter.
- There was mold in the ice machines. Pick a color—green, brown, pink. Yes, mold comes in all of those colors, and one can get hepatitis A, *E. coli*, norovirus, nontyphoidal *Salmonella*, *Salmonella* Typhi, *Shigellosis*, and much more from mold.

Those weren't the only violations, but they were the worst ones.

Ice machines are a pet peeve of mine. They say a picture speaks a thousand words. I will tell you, the mold we health inspectors see is unspeakable. I'm guessing a microbiologist would have a field day identifying the strains of bacteria in many machines. Rarely are they cleaned often enough, if at all. The ice machine in this facility was no exception. (I recently discovered there's no shortage of video clips on TikTok to show you exactly what I am referring to about the ice machines.)

Sometimes restaurant operators don't realize what they're doing is wrong. Other times, they know and, frankly, they don't care. It's evident that they are well aware when they nearly knock you on the floor as they run away with the evidence. That's why we carry a camera.

This facility that I had held in such high esteem had one of the lowest scoring health inspections I have ever conducted. I had dozens of photos and pages of notes. My assistant and I sat down in the restaurant's very dark dining area to complete the inspection form. At the time, everything was handwritten, and we had a significant amount of writing to do.

The owners and one of their children sat at a table near our booth, and it was apparent they were agitated. No one else was in the establishment. I've been in horrific situations throughout my life, and I am not easily intimidated. That irritates people sometimes. I know it did in this situation.

This guy had a reputation for being mentally unstable,
and I had pushed all of his buttons.

With the amount of data we had to contend with, and the dim lighting, it took us quite a while to fill out the report. I knew I was going to close the restaurant. I also knew it was not going to go well.

My assistant and I couldn't discuss anything beyond documenting the information because of the proximity of the owners. The longer it took, the angrier the older gentleman got. They were sitting at a table, and we were in a booth. I kept checking under the table in our booth with my feet to see if it was open enough in case we needed to crawl under it to hide from whatever might come. And I sent a text to my assistant to have 911 ready to dial on her phone.

As this was going on, it was imperative not to look concerned, though we both were. This guy had a reputation for being mentally unstable, and

I had pushed all of his buttons. As we were about to finish the report, the owner sent his wife away, and she hurried out of the dining room.

He said to his son, "Do you remember where I keep the gun?" My assistant and I just looked at each other.

I stood up and said, "Mr. *****, I will be taking your operating license. Please sign this inspection form, and I will leave it here with you. You may reopen after correcting all of the violations and passing a reinspection. Call my office when you are ready, and I will be back."

I turned around, and we briskly walked to the door. I believe we both held our breath the entire way. Once safely outside, I discovered my assistant had also been looking for an escape route as we sat there. When I reviewed the inspection report, I saw that they had accidentally written "casket" instead of "gasket" in the notes. We laughed hysterically, but it had been a dire situation.

This visit was the first of many to this particular restaurant. I left that day with the doors locked behind me and their license in my hand. I was so disappointed. I called the person who oversaw the city's food safety program to tell him what had just happened. This closure would be *big* news, and he needed to know. He met us in the parking lot.

The conversation did not go as I expected. My job was to make sure businesses adhered to state laws and sanitary codes. I took measurements, monitored hygiene and cleanliness, and determined the safety of each location, essentially minimizing risk to the public from foodborne illness. Regardless of who owned the facility, or who its clientele was, public health and safety were my first concern.

Our conversation began like this:

"Do you know who eats here?!" said the person in charge of the city's food safety program.

"I don't care who eats here," I replied angrily. And I'm thinking, *Why does it matter?*

"Every doctor, lawyer, and judge in this town eats in this restaurant!"

"Well, they're damn fortunate they haven't gotten sick, and they can be thankful that someone is doing something about it before they do!" I answered.

"I'm going to get all kinds of flack over this. People aren't going to be happy," he said.

"Tell them to call me, so I can schedule their reinspection when they're ready," I responded.

It was on that day that I decided to get a permit to carry a gun.

Obviously no one in this town had been taking food safety seriously for a very long time. I had had no idea what I was getting into. I think the food safety supervisor thought he had hired a small-town girl who wouldn't pick up on the shenanigans that had been going on. I'm not sure he looked at my credentials.

Rule number one: always do your homework.

And the reinspection didn't go at all well....

NINE

The Reinspection

I got a call saying the fine dining restaurant was ready for reinspection the following day. *Wow, that was fast. They must have called in help and stayed all night. There was so much to do.* That's what I thought.

I was ecstatic the owners had taken the situation seriously. Then again, when you pull someone's operating license off the wall and make them lock their doors, the loss of revenue tends to make them see reality—most of the time.

I was unnerved when I walked into the restaurant kitchen and the staff was (a) preparing to open as if nothing had happened, and (b) the kitchen didn't look any different than it had the day before.

I will never forget him whacking the creature
and briskly sweeping it to the floor...

Plywood shelving still on top of wire shelving—this situation alone was completely unsanitary. Layers of grease on the equipment, food temps inadequate. Was this a joke? To top it off, while I stood beside a counter speaking with the owner—and while he screamed at me for refusing to let him open—a fat cockroach scurried across the countertop where we were standing! I will never forget him whacking the creature and briskly sweeping it to the floor, where he stomped on it.

He may have briefly fantasized it was me.

He did not open that day. It would be one more day before he realized he indeed had to comply with the items in the report or he would not reopen any time soon, and time was money. He had to cancel private events one after another, and frankly, I didn't care.

As all of this transpired, I had repeated flashbacks of a student I had had in a class several years prior. I vividly remembered him telling me about things that went on in a restaurant where he worked. He didn't say where he was employed, but he didn't know that I had a roster that provided me with that information, and of course, I checked. It was this same restaurant.

The student said they'd save uneaten rolls from the tables and reuse them for other diners, or they'd use them for stuffing and croutons (frankly, it wasn't the first time I'd heard of a restaurant doing this). He said the place reserved leftover butter from the tables, because real butter is expensive, right?

And the worst thing he told us? When diners' plates were taken to the kitchen with leftover crab meat or lobster on them, the staff had a "special" place to put those plates. Why? Because they picked the remaining crab and lobster off and used it for things like lobster bisque, cream of crab, chowders, and my favorite—crab au gratin.

But often employees exaggerate, don't they? It couldn't have been as bad as that student said, could it? Surely the health inspector would have picked up on it, or an employee would have called the health department to report something. Of course, none of these thoughts were true, if no one did their job as they should. I had no proof any of the student's stories were true, but I had very little reason to doubt it after the things I saw myself during my visits. If there was a violation to break, this restaurant broke it.

The place was able to open after two days. I guess it finally sunk in that they needed my approval for it to happen.

This may have been our first dance, but it was not our last. This facility continued to stomp on my toes for several years. The owners were horrible individuals who thought they owned the town, and I guess they did have it in their proverbial pocket for years—until I showed up.

Then they didn't know what to do. They had not ever experienced a legitimate health inspection before, at least not in a very long time. Two restaurants in town were very unhappy with me. Brothers owned them. One was the fine dining restaurant I've been discussing, and the other was a very popular diner. I ultimately had to call for police protection when I visited both.

At one point, the fine dining restaurant had a fire in the kitchen, and the fire department had to make an appearance. When that happens, the health inspector has to show up, too. If you've never seen a fire suppression system activate in a restaurant, you don't know what you're missing. It disperses a thin layer of white substance *everywhere*, which can cause chemical contamination if it gets into the food.

Once again, he was livid, and it was my fault.

Any food that is open or uncovered when the system discharges *must* be discarded. It is inedible. But you wouldn't believe the number of individuals who don't or won't acknowledge this...food cost, food cost, food cost.

There's no question that most operators do throw that food away without batting an eye. But there's that small percentage that we had to battle with to make them understand—they are *not* going to use the product. This guy was one of them.

I made him discard all the open food, and he had to wash, rinse, and sanitize all of his dishes and food-contact surfaces before he could reopen after the fire. Once again, he was livid, and it was my fault. Always my fault. He could have opened much sooner if he had started the process right away instead of arguing.

Most of the fire department left, but one guy was still hanging out. Keep in mind the owner had already threatened to shoot me once. At this point, I did have a permit to carry, and this was one of the locations I did not go to anymore without protection. For one place, I needed a police escort to conduct inspections. If I'd had my way, it would have been permanently closed.

After the fire was out that night, we had told the firefighter several times it was okay for him to leave, but he kept wandering around, checking things out. He walked out the door only when we did. We later learned that he was concerned about us. The firefighter didn't want to leave us there alone with the owner after hearing the things he said and seeing how he acted. Our benefactor was afraid the owner would hurt us. He could have gone with the rest of his department, but he chose to stay when he overheard the craziness. What a kind gesture!

Even after all of the inspections I had conducted, this owner thought he could deliver a cease-and-desist letter to stop me from doing health inspections at his facility. I thought I would lose my mind.

I had been doing the inspections for several years by then. I was happy with the improvements I had made in the community's food-service facilities, and my company was growing. Before I received the cease-and-desist letter, I had already decided that I was finished with this part of my career. The guy wasted his money on an attorney. I wasn't returning anyway.

TEN

Cockroaches Keep Falling on My Head

At my foodsafety consulting business, I received a call late one afternoon about an operator who had a severe cockroach infestation. Another health inspector had shut the restaurant down, and the caller needed some direction on how he could most quickly and efficiently get the store up and running again. Closure means loss of income, and time is money.

The voice on the other end of the call asked, "Would you be willing to help?"

"Sure," I replied.

The call had come in from the brand's executive management.

A few minutes later, I got a call from the owner/operator. He had a few questions, the biggest one being: Should he call the PCO right away, or wait until after I came to look things over? I told him to call an exterminator immediately—but not the one he had been using. He needed someone reputable, and I gave him a few names of companies I was familiar with that I knew did an excellent job.

We had a new girl on staff who had recently graduated from college, and I thought this would be an excellent opportunity to train her. I called and asked her to meet me at the facility the following day. I told her to dress professionally but to bring a hooded sweatshirt.

She, of course, asked why.

My response was, "If it's as bad as I expect it will be, it will be raining cockroaches when we get there. You don't want them in your hair, or falling down your shirt."

I was right. Cockroaches fell from the ceiling when we arrived the following day. The new PCO had fumigated the building heavily the evening before, and anything that could breathe was dying in plain sight. We couldn't take a step without hearing the crackle of cockroach shells under our feet. I'm confident this is not what our new hire thought she would be doing when she earned her degree.

Multiple people were here and there in the facility. The owner was floating around with his right-hand man, the store manager was frantic, and employees were trying to clean up the mess. The exterminator was still there from the previous night.

They were floating in the shake machine...

The cockroaches were so nasty and numerous, they were living inside the bearings and legs of the equipment. I realized this when I saw the debris caked on the wheels of various appliances. It got even worse. They were floating in the shake machine, too, as well as inside the warm, dark, moist compressor underneath.

It was a terrible sight. And to think, families with children were eating there just the day before. I thought about this as I watched cockroaches meander through the to-go bags at the frontline counter. Can you imagine reaching into your bag to grab your fries and feeling a cockroach crawl up your hand?!

Over at the fry station, I got down on my hands and knees and saw that the rodent bait station was about two feet away from the wall. Rodent bait stations are supposed to be set tight against a wall. The hole in the trap should be on the side closest to the wall. Remember the song "Three Blind Mice"? Mice don't see well. They use the wall as a guide to get around in a room.

Placing the bait station tight to a wall leads the mice into the trap. I asked the manager to get me a broom. I intended to use the broom handle to push the trap back to its ideal position. But the bait trap stuck to the floor like glue! About an eighth of an inch of crust had built up around the edge of the trap. It would not budge. It apparently had not budged for quite a long time, either.

The facility's right-hand man was standing next to me, along with the manager. The manager was right beside me with a flashlight in her hand. She saw the same thing I saw.

I told the right-hand man to look under the fry station, and he said, "I don't need to."

If I am on my hands and knees in dress clothes under your crappy fry station, with cockroaches falling on my head and crawling under me, your ass can get down here, too.

That's the thought that ran through my brain, not what I said. This man was a *big* guy, over six feet tall and well over two hundred pounds. But I was *not* moving on until he got down and looked at the funk I saw. He should have been checking these things long before I walked in the door.

After he got down on the floor beside me, I started jabbing at the bait station with the broom handle. It took three solid jabs to break that thing loose. I have no idea how long it takes for that much grease to build up and solidify like that, but I believe it's a long time. This situation mortified the store manager, but the right-hand man? He was unfazed.

I noticed the store's employees fluttering about trying to clean up, but not accomplishing much. With a little more observation, I realized no one was giving them any instruction. They did their best to execute what they thought they should.

I approached a young man who was attempting to clean shelves at the front counter. I asked him to get me some soapy water, a green scrubby, and a cloth. He left for a few minutes and returned with the requested supplies. I told him I wanted to help him, and I got down on my knees in front of the shelves to show him how to complete the task.

I stuck my hand in the water, and it was ice cold! I thought, this is my fault—I didn't tell him to get hot water. I assumed he knew.

I said, "I'm sorry. I should have told you. I need hot water."

He replied, "Ma'am, we don't have hot water."

"Excuse me?" I said. I'm thinking, *They've been doing so much cleaning today, maybe they ran out?* Not a chance. I should have known better.

He said, "We don't have a water heater."

I nearly passed out.

"What do you mean you don't have a water heater?" I asked, very dryly.

He casually answered, "It's broken. It hasn't worked for a few days."

OMG, are you kidding me? All of these people have been in this facility working their butts off cleaning up toxic residue with cold water for the last several hours? Everything they'd done had been in vain. An exercise in complete futility.

I was livid. Livid because of the unsanitary conditions. And livid because it was evident that the manager was taking the hit here, and her hands were tied. The magnitude of this situation was not her fault. Livid because these employees were working their butts off unnecessarily. They would have to redo all their work! Livid that there wasn't a damn functional water heater. Livid because the individuals who had control didn't care about any of it. Where the hell was the owner?

The owner showed up at the front counter.

"We need to talk. Let's go outside," I said to him.

"Whatever you have to say, you can say here," he insisted.

"I don't think that's a good idea," I responded. He stood firm.

Okay, have it your way, I thought. I began going through a barrage of issues, and I told him he'd better have hot water there within the next hour or I was calling the corporate office.

He said, "Can we go outside?"

I thought he'd see it my way.

The plumber arrived with a new water heater within thirty minutes. Why did it take that argument to get a new water heater? It should have been common sense—a priority.

But we weren't done yet, for some reason. This facility had a basement. I don't know why. These buildings rarely have a lower level.

But downstairs we went. Who knew what kind of goldmine we'd find down there?

The basement did not disappoint! There stood a freestanding walk-in freezer with so much debris behind it that you could bury an employee back there and no one would ever find them.

We found the largest syrup tank I have ever seen. This thing was massive. Coke syrup was stored in this tank and passed through overhead hoses that carried it to the soda dispensers upstairs. One of the hoses had sprung a leak. The syrup had seeped out onto the floor below and was lying in a large pool around the tank. It had been there long enough to dry out some and become tacky. It was now a glue trap for cockroaches. Hundreds of dead ones were stuck in the syrup.

I left them with seventeen legal-sized pages of notes on things they would have to do to reopen.

And cockroaches weren't the only issue. I could see tiny mouse prints all through the syrup, too. I shined my UV light on it, and it glowed like a nuclear waste dump—rodent urine glows under UV light.

We spent hours in the facility that day. It was a Saturday, their busiest weekend of the year, and they would not open any time soon. I left them with seventeen legal-sized pages of notes on things they would have to do to reopen.

When I was finally done, I had to call their corporate office from the parking lot. The executive asked me if they'd be able to open the next day.

I laughed out loud and said: "Have you ever been here?"

Her response was, "Will you please go back on Monday?"

My job was to get them open as quickly, efficiently, and inexpensively as possible. I was up for a challenge, but I am not a miracle worker.

On my way home—a three-hour drive—I stopped on the turnpike, changed my clothes, and threw everything I was wearing away, including my shoes. If you tramp on a pregnant cockroach, you can carry the eggs back home in the tread of your shoes.

On Monday, the place showed significant improvement. They had fogged the store twice with three times the legal limit of the chemical solution, but roaches were still alive. I swear these things will survive a nuclear holocaust. The owner didn't want to throw his paper products away, even though they were covered in toxic residue.

This resulted in another heated discussion. Why do people insist on saving money at the expense of other people's lives?

I couldn't eat at their facilities for a very long time. The psychological repercussions were too great.

In some cases, these facilities are found in malls or strip malls, and the insects travel about the building, running from one store to another. That was not the case here. This place was a freestanding facility. These situations are blamed on a multitude of things. The neighboring buildings, vendors, employees, customers, etc. The infestations don't always arise because of cleanliness issues, but they do persist due to poor cleaning habits. The roaches moved in and continued to reside in this freestanding facility because of the filth and grime and lack of treatment. Not because they were moving about a larger environment seeking food and shelter.

The store opened on Wednesday of that week with zero violations. The health inspector and executive management were amazed, as was I. To this day, this place is one of the worst facilities I have ever seen. There is no excuse—*none*—for an owner to allow a facility to deteriorate to this condition.

But I know this brand well. I have worked for them in several capacities and know this is not their standard. I've done inspections for them, trained for them, and consulted with them. That was just a terrible owner/operator. Even though I knew that was the case, and the place was far from the norm for the brand, I couldn't eat at their facilities for a very long time. The psychological repercussions were too great.

I had "character" hardwood floors with dark knots in them at home. Sometimes I would catch a glimpse of a knot out of the corner of my eye, or a piece of brown fuzz on the floor, and I'd experience a significant moment of panic. It took a year or more for that to go away.

The experience was one of the most impactful of my career, and one I will never forget.

ELEVEN

Oh, Rats!

What happens when the pest control operator can't gain control of a rodent infestation within city limits? They call the health department for enforcement.

Unfortunately, rats had overtaken a quaint downtown, ordinarily a charming area. On the surface, everything appeared to be as one would expect. A six-tiered fountain with flowing water in the town square, flowers planted along the street, restaurants with alfresco dining, birds chirping, and people meandering in and out of the local shops. But there was another part to this town that most folks didn't know about, and frankly, I wish I didn't, either.

The buildings on each block downtown are connected underground, with doors in their foundations to separate one property from another. People, rodents, and various other creatures can move freely about the entire neighborhood—over walls, through cracks, and under and through doors.

When an infestation of any type occurs, if all affected residents don't work together to schedule pest control treatments, the problem is virtually impossible to control or eliminate. Let's say building 100 gets treated. The insects and rodents will relocate to buildings 99 and 101, where no treatment has happened yet. Then when the PCO treats buildings 99 and 101, those same insects and rodents pack up and come back to building 100. It's a vicious cycle. The ideal solution is for the

PCO to treat buildings 99, 100, and 101 simultaneously on the same rotation. Get them coming and going.

Rats have long cylindrical bodies that are flexible, allowing them to jam their bodies through small holes. They do have bones! There is no truth to the rumor that they do not. But mice can fit through a hole the size of a dime, and rats can squeeze through a space the size of a quarter. Yes, you read that right—the size of a quarter!

Rats breed so quickly, too, that in just eighteen months, two rats can produce enough generations to number over one *million* relatives, and they can produce nearly one *billion* in three years. Imagine how quickly they can take over an abandoned building if they have food and water.

Forget using that spray foam around your pipes. It's a snack.

Rats are athletes, too. They can lunge three feet in the air, can climb up just about anything, and can swim half a mile at a stretch. I've seen rats scale concrete-block walls. They can even climb or swim up the inside of pipes and survive a fifty-foot drop.

Rats will eat almost anything, including poop and trash. The Smithsonian National Zoo reported that one rat they studied had more than 4,000 unique materials in its stomach. They can also chew through almost anything non-metallic—their teeth grow continuously throughout their lives, so gnawing helps keep their teeth sharp and trimmed. Forget using that spray foam around your pipes. It's a snack. Use a metal covering to seal openings and keep these intruders out.

Knowing this bit of information about these rodents will give you a clear perspective on my assignment. The PCO was tasked with getting the "rodent situation" under control in this little town. But he had no authority there. Many affected locations had owners who wouldn't agree to pay for PCO services. So, of course, he couldn't provide the required services.

The borough council had to call the health department (me) for enforcement. I was not excited about this. As always, though, I showed up with a smile on my face—and the rest of me defended by the tallest pair of leather boots I could find, a hat, a heavy jacket, and jeans. If the rats attacked me, I'd make them work for it.

Did I mention there was no light in these underground passageways between all these buildings?

As soon as we hit the bottom step at the first location, I could hear the rustling and squeaking noises one would expect to hear from an army of rats. I had a hat on, but not a hard hat. I hoped my hat was enough because, while I knew they're physically skilled and coordinated, I still expected our presence to scare the rats crawling on the rafters above our heads, and they'd fall, or worse yet, lunge at me.

The PCO had a flashlight. I had my notepad and pen. Movement on the rafters overhead was undeniable. My skin crawled. There was ample evidence of rodent infestation everywhere, including feces, urine, rodent tracks, and dead rat carcasses. It was important to me not to let my fears become evident on my face or in my voice as I listened to these noises and tramped over dead rat remains during the evaluation.

It didn't take long to forward my report confirming that there was indeed a rodent infestation in the area the town had inquired about, and PCO enforcement was necessary—pronto!

I will never forget the feelings I had that day. I had known it would be an experience unlike any other, but I had had no idea how many rats there would be. I had known it would be enough to create a bona fide infestation issue, but this was like a horror movie. I was not mentally prepared for it.

My anxiety level spiraled higher than I had ever experienced. I thought my heart would explode through my chest, and my skin itched so badly I expected to break out in hives at any second. I hope never to experience anything like this again.

As I went in and out of restaurants in the downtown neighborhood, the rodent issue was evident everywhere. Large bait stations were placed around almost every facility. Exterminators only used these large traps for rats, not mice. Occasionally, I'd see a rat scurry by, and they were huge. I swear you could saddle them.

It was apparent which facilities didn't use a PCO, because they were using gigantic wooden rat traps. The last thing I wanted to encounter that day was a rat freshly caught in one of those traps, attempting to make its escape.

Even though they knew they had a problem, some of the establishments I needed to inspect did not welcome me with open arms. I didn't realize they'd object when I set out on this task. Sadly, this wasn't all that unusual through my entire time as an inspector.

I felt more feared than the dentist! God bless dentists.

I've always been one to say yes to a project and figure the details out later. I wish I had thought this through on the rat detail. The problem was I assumed everyone was like me. When I managed restaurants, I looked forward to visits from the health inspector. I saw them as a challenge. They allowed me to prove that I was doing a good job—validation, I suppose.

Unfortunately, too many operators don't feel the same. They see sanitarians as the devil out to get them and cause trouble, not someone who protects their business and public health. Even the operators doing a good job don't necessarily care for the health inspector. I felt more feared than the dentist! God bless dentists.

I always saw myself as there to help establishments learn and grow, not as an adversary. Even in dire situations, I tried to work with operators as best I could, as long as they weren't threatening or hostile toward me. Part of the problem during the rat infestation was that too many operations hadn't been inspected in so long—years—and they didn't understand the sudden change in how their health department conducted business. It was confusing for them, I'm sure. I understood, and I tried to be sensitive to their situation.

Most of the facilities I ever inspected had nothing to worry about, because they were doing a good job. But about 20 percent of them regularly wreaked havoc on my life. I never told anyone about a violation without explaining how to fix it. I wanted to work with them, but it had to be mutual. I couldn't fix their problems for them.

It took over a year to get most of those downtown businesses on board and get the rats moved out. But that was only one problem I dealt with in that place. Bootleg foods was another. The operators were always trying to convince me I was crazy. Every time I walked into one facility, there'd be homemade pie on the counter beside the cash register, with a missing slice or two.

They'd tell me, "It's for us. We ate it. Aunt ***** made it. Want a piece? It's so good!"

Next door, they'd have gallon canning jars of peppers in the back room, about seventy of them! "For *home*!" they'd say.

Children's toys would be strewn all over the floor and a playpen set up in a storage area where a few adorable children played. Regulatory authorities frown on children playing in the kitchen at foodservice facilities, and this was a definite violation.

I was a human being before I was a health inspector...

It took some time, but we came to an understanding. If they'd just stop doing these other things, they could stay open, but they could *not* sell food products that are home-canned.

A block or so down from that facility, I found a gentleman making homemade tortilla shells in a highly unique bowl. As I watched, I realized it was a slice of a tree that had been used for so long, it had been worn down to a bowl shape.

I was 100 percent certain the "bowl" was not acceptable for a commercial kitchen. This is the type of situation that can get tricky. I was a human being before I was a health inspector, and while 99.9 percent of the time that does not affect my job, there are moments when it does. This was one of those moments. There was no chance I would force this man to throw the bowl away. He had brought it to the United States from his homeland. It had been his father's before him.

But he did have to get it out of the store. I let him take it to his car and told him if I found it in his kitchen again, he would have to throw it in the dumpster. My reputation had preceded me, and he knew

I meant it. He would not bring the bowl back. I can't begin to tell you how appreciative he was. Yes, it was a clear violation and written up as one. But to make him destroy that piece of wood would have been vicious, in my opinion—a power play.

TWELVE

Intentional Deception

After visiting several restaurants owned by the same family in one town, I noticed that the food manager certifications were held by people with exactly the same name. I know in certain ethnicities it is common for many people in the family to share a name, and some specific first names become trendy.

But for that to be the name of every individual with a food manager certification in each restaurant? That's not likely. Since recording this information was part of my standard inspection process, catching it didn't take long. I realized it was time to investigate.

> Unfortunately, some operators see the certificate
> as an unnecessary burden on their business.

I went to each facility and took a photo of their food manager certification so I could validate the information. These certificates are essential: they certify that someone in the facility has passed an exam and has the bare minimum food safety knowledge required. Unfortunately, some operators see the certificate as an unnecessary burden on their business. Getting one incurs an additional day or two away from work for the PICs and the expense of learning materials. And, of course, turnover in the industry is high, so recertifying someone new creates even more cost.

The certificates have multiple identifying dates and numbers associated with each one, like exam date, expiration date, and certificate number. It's easy to identify fraud.

Sure enough, all of these owners had made a copy of one certificate, all the dates and numbers the same, and hung the copies in their restaurants so it appeared they were meeting the local regulations.

In their jurisdiction, a foodservice operation cannot hold a license to operate unless they comply with all the health and safety regulations. A facility may lose its liquor license, and they're hard to come by. Excellent reasons to follow the guidelines—but I had found several who did not.

I could tell by the expiration date on the certificate that this certification game had been going on for some time. Imagine their surprise when I figured it out so quickly. Their first response was to say that they all had the same name. Okay, fine, I get it, my son is named after his father. "But I need you to explain how you all have identical certificate numbers." Crickets.

You wouldn't believe the number of restaurants I've discovered over the years that operated without a license.

Several members of the owning family were not happy with me. Many considered the food safety class useless and a waste of their time. But that didn't matter. They had thirty days to make a legal certificate happen, meaning not only did they need to schedule an exam, but they needed to pass it, as well.

You wouldn't believe the number of restaurants I've discovered over the years that operated without a license. I'd be driving down the street and see a place that I didn't recall seeing on the list of operations in my jurisdiction. So I'd check. Sure enough, not on the list, but there it was, open for business. Ninety-nine percent of the time, that meant they never got a license to operate. I'd pay a visit. The first thing I'd do is ask to see their operating permit, and, of course, they wouldn't have one. One guy ran out the back door and left me standing there.

There is an established process for getting a permit to open a food-service operation, but these folks just set up and opened their doors without bothering. Can you imagine? I was appalled at some of these situations. I can't fathom the thought of opening any establishment without going through the proper channels.

I am willing to help anyone out, bend over backward, do cartwheels if I have to. But I will not tolerate intentional deception and people lying to me. That takes things to an entirely different level. It's something we don't quickly recover from, if ever.

Take, for instance, telling me your meat products are all USDA certified, when I just caught you slaughtering a goat in your kitchen. And you don't have invoices for meat purchases. That's a bold-faced lie. I won't trust this person—not ever.

One week, we had someone scheduled to teach a local food manager class. Restaurant owners don't realize I own the company conducting that class, and if I just confirmed that they told me a lie, I was not likely to believe anything they told me. The people who butchered the goat knew that I knew that they weren't telling the truth—they couldn't provide a registration paper for the product.

"I just put those in the cooler and haven't had time to put a date on them yet," someone would say. I stand there looking at the product, and I can see that the grease is solidified and the product beside it isn't even recognizable. Epic fail.

Sometimes I had to shake my head in disbelief. On one particular day, I had saved the "easiest" location for last. But if there is one thing I have learned over the years, it's never assume anything—*ever*. This inspection was no exception. The establishment was a small coffee shop. They served coffee, tea, and a few select pastries. That's it. They knew I was in the building by the time I got to their location. The inspection that should have taken twenty or thirty minutes took over an hour.

Everything derailed when I asked to see their temperature log. Temperature logs are a big deal in the foodservice business. In this case, if they didn't have their temperature logs accurately completed for the last thirty days, they'd fail the inspection regardless of how well they had performed on the rest of the assessment. This was a third-party review, and that was company policy.

As I looked through the temperature logs, this is what I noticed:

- The same person was listed as taking the temperatures on all three shifts, seven days a week, all month.
- They used the same writing utensil for every single entry.
- Not one temperature was out of range for the entire month.
- There was no missed logging, and no temperatures were taken late in thirty days.
- The pages on the temperature log were pristine—not one drop of tea, coffee, or water, not one bent corner, nothing.

Clearly a case of falsifying company documentation—and grounds for immediate termination. When the operators heard I was in the facility, the PIC went through all the pertinent logs and filled them out as though someone had completed them during the month. She would have been better off leaving them blank. Failing to keep the logs was less of a problem than falsifying them. If you work in the foodservice industry, a word to the wise: do not do this, *ever.*

The people who do inspections and audits will know, and you will lose your job. It's not worth it.

THIRTEEN

The Perceived Enemy

After several months of working as the health inspector, I'd wake up in the morning and my first thought would be, "Dear God, please let it be a good day."

I don't believe there is a health inspector out there who enjoys closing restaurants. It takes a lot of time and effort to deal with shutting someone down. You don't do it on a whim.

First, there is the stress and drama involved in telling the owner/operator that they need to close because they are not operating their business as required for health and safety. No one operating a food-service facility thinks for a second that they don't know precisely what they are doing and how to do it.

Second, there is a tremendous amount of paperwork involved in shutting them down. This isn't something that can be done simply because you have the urge to shut down a restaurant on a particular day. When an inspector decides to close a restaurant, they better make damn sure they have sufficient documentation to do it.

Third, once it's been closed down, the facility must pass a complete inspection to reopen. So when an inspector closes a facility, it means they need to fit another health inspection into their already overbooked schedule, and the operation must pass that inspection before it's allowed to reopen. Typically this reinspection goes well (not always), but at that point the inspector is the perceived enemy, the one who closed them in the first place. It's not a pleasant experience, but it goes with the territory. Sometimes you walk into a place and there might be five or six executives following you around, taking notes while you do your job. Occasionally it may be an owner and his attorney(s).

Fourth, we are human beings, and shutting someone's business down takes an emotional toll. I knew that closing an establishment sometimes meant these folks would have no income, but the bills would still accumulate. Maybe the manager would be terminated. I did not take that lightly. The position of a health inspector is not for the meek or the weak.

I do love my job. I always have. Training and educating people and sharing my knowledge excites me. There's a difference between those two aspects. It is essential to show someone how to do a job *and* tell them why they are doing it. Showing is training; explaining is educating.

Many foodborne illnesses cause potentially lifelong ramifications, or maybe even death.

The best analogy I can give is: Should children have sex training or sex education? I believe the answer is obvious. Education is important.

In the early years of my restaurant career, my manager always told us we must put raw chicken on the bottom shelf, but no one ever told me why. As a result, I usually put it on the bottom shelf. But if there wasn't space, I might occasionally have placed it over the produce. I don't know, but it's possible.

That manager should have included the information that if juices (aka blood) from raw chicken drip down on a ready-to-eat food like salad veggies, and someone eats those vegetables, various illnesses can result. Bacteria such as *Salmonella* Typhi or *Campylobacter jejuni* often reside in chicken drippings. *Campylobacter* can lead to Guillain-Barré syndrome and reactive arthritis. *Salmonella* infections can lead to meningitis, endocarditis, and osteomyelitis. Many foodborne illnesses cause potentially lifelong ramifications, or maybe even death.

Knowing all that—I would never put chicken where it can drip on other foods! Why didn't anyone ever provide me with this knowledge when I was starting out? I assure you it would have factored into my decisions.

In the United States alone, 48 million people (that's 1 in 6!) contract foodborne diseases each year, 128,000 are hospitalized, and *3,000 die every year* from food poisoning. Globally, 600 million (1 in 10) people fall ill, and 420,000 people die from eating contaminated food. And what's even more shocking is that these are all 100 percent preventable!

All of these illnesses happen because someone, somewhere in the food chain, screwed up—they didn't do their job. Sometimes prevention is as simple as food handlers washing their hands. A person can spread many of these illnesses through the fecal-oral route—with a very small amount of contamination—and one person can therefore sicken many people.

A person with a contagious illness that's transmitted through the fecal-oral route uses the restroom, doesn't wash their hands adequately, and opens the bathroom door. The person behind them washes their hands well, but opens the same contaminated door, and then picks something out from between their teeth or anxiously bites their nails before washing their hands again.

Bing, bang, boom, that microbe has now been spread through the fecal-oral route.

If the individual who picks up contamination works in a kitchen, they will spread it to everything they handle, including the gloves they put on their hands, the produce they put on sandwiches, or the point-of-sale terminal where they check out purchases. It's a disaster waiting to happen, and it does—every day. No one should ever die from eating food.

Always wash your hands and use a new, clean paper towel to touch the faucet handles and open the door!

My decision to write this book came about because, one day, I made a decision to protect the health of the public, and people literally turned on me right before my eyes. It happened unexpectedly and very quickly. I had a wide array of emotions in a very short time, and it's hard to even begin to explain. One second, I was doing my job. The next, I was protecting an employee, and I was worried about her safety and my own.

I went from wanting to do my job to keep some people from consuming harmful substances, to wanting to shove the food down their throats—literally. I am not a violent person, not even close, but the things that happened at that moment were so unbelievable, I felt like I was in a scene from some movie. All it took was one vocal leader for things to spiral out of control, and out of control they went. I can tell you, I haven't looked at bacon the same since, and the incident happened a decade ago.

More on that later....

FOURTEEN

Choices Are Decisions That Can Impact Us Acutely

I traveled across the United States and back again for several years working for a national corporation. I was one of the few trainers the company used, and I loved working with their team. They had the kindest employees, who were always prepared for class, and wanted to do a good job. I am also a regular consumer of their brand, and I have done multiple health inspections in their facility. Talk about perspective.

As a consumer, I always notice that their common areas are clean, neat, and orderly. The employees are well groomed and tidy, their uniforms are consistent, and they're friendly and polite. The stores are clean, the parking lots are clean, and their sign is always well lit and all of the bulbs work.

Yes, I do notice all of this. That comes from years of working in the business and in my current career, and it comes naturally. I just take notice.

A few years ago, my husband and I were sitting in the airport in Mexico, and I was looking up at the ceiling. We were just passing the time waiting for our flight, but he looked at me rather strangely and asked, "What are you doing?"

"Counting burned-out light bulbs," I laughed. I honestly didn't even realize I was doing it until he pointed it out. Years as a professional in this industry will do that to you.

My point to this story is that I traveled to these stores all over the United States, and the brand was consistent. Sure, everyone has a bad day, and there might be a renegade or two, but I speak of nearly two thousand locations—consistent. I always wonder why their competitor can't (doesn't) do the same thing. I mean, they're hiring from the same demographic. It's ultimately a choice they make.

Sometimes, right or wrong, I would mention these observations in my classes. It was my justified observation.

When my granddaughter was five years old, I needed to make a pit stop for her to use a restroom. As we stopped and headed into said competitor's facility, she said, "Nanny, please not here. Wherever we stop, their bathrooms are always dirty, and they smell!"

Even she noticed. I glanced behind me, and two employees were about four steps behind us. I was mortified. Five-year-olds have no filter.

My daughter deemed the bathroom there too filthy to use.

But she was right. We turned around, and I took her somewhere else. As we walked to the car, I remembered a time her mother was about the same age, and she refused to use a restroom. We were on vacation and had stopped for gas. My daughter deemed the bathroom there too filthy to use. We went someplace else then, too. When they're right, they're right. Observations and perceptions begin at a very young age.

Choices people make, like thinking it's acceptable to turn off their water heater during the lunch rush to save money or operating without clean water, truly puzzle me. It is not okay.

Choices are ultimately decisions that can impact people acutely for a long time.

Employees or customers can't wash their hands, and it is impossible to wash dishes or clean and sanitize the facility without water—clean, hot water. We had one restaurant that would shut this off regularly.

One day right after lunch, I walked into a popular pizza restaurant. The facility was immaculate, though short-staffed. They had just had a killer lunch rush. I began my inspection by taking temperatures at the prep station. As soon as I lifted the lid on the station, I could smell the stench. It was awful.

I tend to want to give people the benefit of the doubt, so I initially wondered if it could be my imagination, even though I knew 100 percent without a doubt it was not. It was always a fleeting thought to wonder, but it happened.

I immediately began taking temperatures, thinking, *How could someone not smell this?!* The table was right beside the pizza oven, only a few feet away. Items in the prep table are supposed to be stored at less than 41°F, and the pizza oven is at least 800°F. The proximity of these two pieces of equipment alone creates an issue, but I was sure there was more of a problem.

Potentially Hazardous Foods—now called Time/Temperature Controlled for Safety (TCS) foods—are defined in the Food Code as foods most likely to cause a foodborne illness outbreak. None of the TCS items in this restaurant were within the safe range, and everything was higher than room temperature. I began to feel sick in my stomach, knowing how many pizzas they had just sold over lunch.

I asked to see the temperature log, and there wasn't one. I inquired how long the items had been in the prep cooler. The employee told me they had been there since the previous night. They hadn't put them away in the walk-in cooler.

I didn't know if this had been an issue for two hours, four hours, ten hours, or longer, but it didn't matter. It was a severe problem, and this was a national brand. Why does that matter? Because their protocol for handling these situations is different from the process for an independent restaurant. First, they *have* a protocol for this event, and many independents don't. It's irrelevant to an inspector, but the employee had to make a few calls immediately. At that point, the average inspector would have left her and her company to deal with the issues, but I believe in helping to educate and solve problems when I can.

They closed the store because they didn't have any additional staff or prep to put on the table. The district manager was due to arrive any minute. We pulled the prep table away from the wall. It was turned on, and the breakers were on, but we found the plug lying on the floor. It appeared that when the staff cleaned up the night before, they'd pulled the table out too far and it had unplugged. Mystery solved.

Those items sat in the prep table all the previous night and half the day with no refrigeration. Ground beef, chicken, sausage, ham, bacon, mushrooms, chicken wings, and more were on that prep table, and they had sold nearly two hundred pizzas over lunch. The prep station, boxing area, and working tools were all close by and could have been contaminated. A recipe for disaster.

I was sure we would be flooded with complaints, but we didn't receive one. I always wondered how many people got sick and thought they had the flu. We will never know.

Had the person working that day made the choice to take the temperature of items in the prep station as recommended, all the problems that followed could have been avoided. Choices are decisions. Good or bad, there are consequences. Not taking the temperatures of the food products when that person arrived resulted in the following:

- Serving food that had been at room temperature for an excessive amount of time, thus reaching the point of spoilage in some cases,
- The possibility of customers becoming ill from eating the food that was sold,
- Not realizing the prep table was unplugged,
- Closure of the restaurant for a few hours,
- Possible disciplinary action,
- Potential litigation,
- Media attention, and
- Lost sales.

These are just a few of the consequences of her poor decision. The entire scenario would have been much different if she had just done her job, which would have been to take the product temperatures and then perform corrective action when she discovered a problem.

Throw the inferior product away. Find the root cause of the problem—here, the unplugged prep table. Plug the prep table in and make sure it's working properly. Wash, rinse, and sanitize the entire table inside and out. Then put fresh product on the table in clean prep pans.

Bing, bang, boom! When the health inspector shows up, everything is working properly and it's a wonderful day in the neighborhood. The consequences would have been entirely different.

FIFTEEN

What Is in That Box?

Running my company—including consulting, training, and doing third-party inspections—meant traveling nationally several days a week, with a bit of international travel, as well. When my company was sub-contracted to conduct municipal health inspections on top of all that, it didn't take long before I was exhausted, both mentally and physically.

At first I conducted well over two hundred inspections a year, but that number snowballed quickly, with reinspections, emergencies, complaints, new facility openings, and special events all adding to the mix.

These additions amounted to about a hundred extra inspections annually, too much for one person to handle. I developed a plan to organize the additional inspections more efficiently, and I eventually hired someone to help me with the inspections. Having a new inspector on board would be incredible, but I was hoping the demands wouldn't be too much for him. His first training day on the job, I met my new hire at the local Starbucks. He was someone I knew and had worked with previously. We covered a few details and headed to our first stop.

We walked in the door, introduced ourselves, showed the owner our IDs, and headed to the kitchen. The facility had a "pass-through" cooler-freezer in the kitchen, which means you had to walk through the cooler to get to the freezer—all very routine, until I opened the freezer door.

Inspectors must capture a snapshot of a typical day at a facility when they conduct an inspection. That's why these visits are unannounced. What good would it do if everyone had time to prep for their health inspection? If that was the case and anyone's inspection was less than perfect, that would be an absolute disgrace. Not to mention wondering what they might do the other 363 days when the inspector wasn't coming (we inspected twice a year).

There was no question this facility did not expect us. I opened the freezer door a few inches and thought I must have imagined what I saw inside. I slowly closed it.

My trainee said, "Francine, are you OK?"

The owner tried to push past my trainee, who was rapidly snapping photos for evidence.

I replied, "Yes. You're not going to believe this." Now, remember, this was his first day. I didn't want him to run out the back door screaming like his hair was on fire, but we were about to enter into a precarious situation.

I opened the door again, and we stepped inside the freezer. There were half a dozen hooved legs strewn about the floor. To my right was a box containing a black trash bag folded out over the edge. Another hooved leg peeked out over the edge of the box. The lid was raised just a bit, and I could immediately tell that the container was filled with something else that shouldn't be in it—I just wasn't sure what it was.

I looked at the box, thinking, *What is in that box? I don't want to open the box. I have to open the box. OH. MY. GOD. I don't want to open that box. OK, let's do this.* I lifted the top.

Now this is all happened very quickly—all in less than a minute. I reached for the box's lid, and as I lifted it, the owner tried to push past my trainee, who was rapidly snapping photos for evidence.

My trainee was a large fellow, tall and stocky. The owner didn't get past him in time, and I got the box open. Inside were baby goats—*carcasses of baby goats.* They had just finished slaughtering them in the kitchen before we walked in the door. Oy vey!

Apparently, they had trouble gathering up the legs quickly enough, and they ended up strewn all over the freezer floor.

That operating license was off the wall in about thirty seconds. That's how long it took to walk over to the wall where it was hanging. We had them lock their doors. I was praying my trainee would finish day one and return for day two.

Welcome to my world.

We were fifteen minutes into the day, and I thought I'd brought him to a location that would be safe, easy. The kitchen wasn't supposed to be a makeshift butcher shop with black market baby goats in the freezer.

"It's for home use," they said.

"I don't believe you," I said. "You have goat on the menu. I do not see any USDA-inspected goat in the freezer."

"We are out," he said.

I said, "Then we have another problem, because you're selling something on the buffet labeled goat."

They could not produce any invoices for USDA-inspected goat meat, either. The owner called his attorney, threatened litigation, and told me his invoices were at home in another state. I told him I would meet him the following morning, and if he had the appropriate paperwork, he could reopen.

This gentleman should not have been operating
a restaurant under any circumstances.

It wasn't the sort of day I had planned.

I showed up at the restaurant early the next day. The owner was forty-five minutes late. He had a few handwritten invoices from a supplier that I could not verify and a few additional invoices from what would be considered an approved supplier, dated many, many months prior. It appeared he had been using "fresh farm goats" for a while.

This gentleman should not have been operating a restaurant under any circumstances. Many of the folks I inspected should have been closed permanently, fined, and potentially faced with jail time. None of that ever happened.

The bottom line is that the person who'd been running the health department wasn't qualified. That's how the previous inspector got away with the things she did (nepotism was also at play, as were calling ahead to announce inspections, stopping in only to get the inspection form signed, or not even inspecting at all but filling out the forms and submitting them anyway). Many of the establishments in that jurisdiction went years without an inspection.

The operators *loved* the previous inspector! Many of them despised me, and they didn't hesitate to share that information with me or anyone else who would listen.

I don't believe the person in charge of the local health department did his research before hiring me. We lived in the same small town, and I'm confident he thought he hired a small-town girl who wouldn't make waves and wasn't as knowledgeable as I am. I don't know if he didn't understand the term "subject matter expert," or if he thought I was kidding when I told him that's what I am. I'm better known on the national stage than in my local community for my expertise in food safety and food safety advocacy. The guy who hired me bit off way more than he could chew, and there was nothing he could do about it. I was creating more headaches than he or anyone else in a position of authority over the health department wanted to deal with with. C'est la vie.

SIXTEEN

The Night I Sat in My Car and Cried

I clearly remember the one day I felt defeated. Not because my job didn't get done, or done correctly, but because sometimes people are just victims of circumstance.

That doesn't change the parameters or the importance of my job, or mean I should alter how I do it. It simply makes it more emotionally complicated for me, because even though health inspectors shouldn't show it when we're in a facility, sometimes the situations rip our hearts out.

I believe that happens in many careers.

They had mounded the semi-frozen chicken pieces
far above the rim.

I was inspecting a very popular all-you-can-eat buffet restaurant. This place had a huge list of health code violations and fire code violations, as well. The first thing that caught my eye was the kitchen sink. Restaurants are typically required to have three-bay sinks intended for dishwashing, set up for wash, rinse, and sanitize. Not only was this one grotesque from afar, but it was filled with frozen chicken that was thawing at room temperature. There must have been five or six cases of chicken in the first bay, at forty pounds each. They had mounded the semi-frozen chicken pieces far above the rim. The other two sink bays were filled with dirty dishes.

My next observation was off to my right, where the vents in their exhaust hood over the grill had a thick syrupy liquid on it that dripped down onto food being prepared for the buffet. To my left, an employee was washing dishes in a mop sink beside a dirty mop bucket.

Everyone in the kitchen was in a panic, chattering and scurrying about as I snapped pictures. It was total sensory overload.

What the hell is happening here?

That was one of many thoughts that ran through my head. At this point, I hadn't been in the facility for three minutes yet. Who knew what else I would find? All I knew was, this would likely take hours, and it wouldn't be pleasant.

My assistant and I started work in a back corner of the facility, finding one priority violation after another:

- Employees not washing their hands,
- Improper cooking procedures,
- Improper reheating procedures,
- Improper cooling procedures,
- Improper holding temperatures for hot and cold food items,
- Improper thawing procedures,
- Raw meat products stored over ready-to-eat food,
- Cockroaches in the soft-serve machine and in every other device in the facility,
- Piles of roaches in every corner of the kitchen,
- Children playing in the kitchen, and…
- …the list went on and on.

They needed to close the restaurant.

My assistant and I had been in the facility for a while at this point. We wore white lab coats, took temperatures, and wrote notes on a clipboard.

As the owner locked the doors and put a "CLOSED" sign in the window, a gentleman walked up to us and asked, "Do we have to leave? Is it okay if we finish our meal?"

Let me give you a tip: if you see someone in an official white lab coat taking temperatures, and suddenly the owner of the restaurant you're eating in locks the doors, put your fork down and go home. Can you finish your meal? Sure. Should you? I would not.

As it turned out, the owners of this facility did not speak much English. They were one of the most popular restaurants in town, and I'm sure they'd been operating like this for years. It wasn't possible for all of these issues to accumulate overnight, or even in six months.

I needed to sit down with them to go over the inspection, and it was a multi-page report. By the time I'd been there for five hours, they were terrified, and I was exhausted and upset—as much with my predecessor as with the owners.

Going over the inspection took more than two more hours.

When we sat down to discuss the issues, two young children appeared at the side of the table. It took me a second to realize what was happening. The parents were at the table, visibly upset. The children, who had arrived after school and played in the kitchen, were overwhelmed and upset to see their parents' demeanor. I was responsible for upsetting Mom and Dad, and the kids were there to translate what I was about to say.

They were a girl and a boy, approximately six and eight years old, respectively. How could I relate to these young children the depth and seriousness of the issues here?

I do not want to do this!

Honestly, I wanted nothing more than to pack my stuff up and go home. These children looked devastated, my empathy-meter was off the charts, and my mom-heart was breaking.

The language barrier made it an even more challenging situation. The children sometimes struggled with the translation, and I wonder if it was partly because they felt the information they had to relay to their parents was disrespectful coming from them. Going over the inspection took more than two more hours. I had gotten to the restaurant around nine that morning and didn't leave until eight that evening. A long day.

But it was important to me that they understood precisely what they needed to accomplish, and that I didn't leave the family in shambles.

I walked out, sat in my car, and cried.

Such a disservice had been done to these people over the past several years. Many of us would know that most of what was happening was wrong, especially the cleanliness issues. But you don't know what no one has ever taught you. And what those children had just experienced—not my fault, but I'm still a mother.

My heart broke for them and their parents on a personal level. If I ever felt less than human for doing my job, it was that night. But there were so many severe violations in that facility that I honestly couldn't imagine that no one ever got sick. I am sure people did, and assumed they had the flu.

I have since overheard people say they ate there and became ill. Being the expert in the room and making certain the restaurant owners complied with food safety rules, while they stood shaking in front of me, was horrific. I know I did the right thing, but it didn't make me feel any better on a personal level.

SEVENTEEN

She's a Bitch on a Power Trip

It was the weekend, a beautiful summer weekend. Honestly, the last thing I wanted to do was health inspections, but a fishing rodeo for kids and a few other special events were happening, so off I went. Even though it was not what I wanted to do, I wasn't angry or upset about it. I intended to get to the sites, dive in, get the work done, and get home. An easy day.

How many times have I made that assumption?

The same people who weighed and measured the fish were smoking cigars.

My first stop proved otherwise. This location was where the children brought their freshly caught fish to be measured and weighed. They were excited and having a blast. It was fun to watch them as they brought their trout up to the scales.

At the same site, the group was holding your typical fundraiser, selling hamburgers, hot dogs, chips, and beverages. None of this was a big deal, except they had no water to wash their hands, no hand soap, no single-use gloves, and no hand sanitizer.

The same people who weighed and measured the fish were smoking cigars, handling raw ground beef and hot dogs, and preparing sandwiches. With no water, or soap, or gloves.

So this was my visual: men weighing freshly caught fish, handling raw meat, placing cooked meat on buns, and serving them—all while smoking cigars!

I thought I was on *Candid Camera*. I think I blacked out for a few moments. This was mind blowing.

I immediately addressed them, and they were not happy. They informed me this had been their procedure for years and "ain't nobody got sick yet," and they didn't need me to tell them what to do.

Unfortunately for them, I was in charge, and I had a problem with their system.

The remaining gentlemen stood behind me—unkindly—
whining and complaining.

I pulled the person running the event aside and kindly explained my concerns and what needed to be corrected immediately. They needed to find a way to wash their hands with soap and warm water and get some single-use gloves. Pronto. As I explained this, the remaining gentlemen stood behind me—unkindly—whining and complaining.

I made some suggestions to the PIC as to where he might find the tools he needed to become compliant.

I gave them forty-five minutes to remedy the problems, or I would have to close the entire food operation. There were multiple violations and risk factors. Foodborne illnesses are no joke. I looked around the site, choosing my battles. *E. coli*, norovirus, hepatitis A, and Staph were my biggest concerns. They were only permitted to sell beverages and chips during those forty-five minutes. I was more than kind. Just do it.

As I walked away, I heard one of the gentlemen (I use the term loosely) say, "She's a bitch on a power trip."

I promptly turned around, said, "I'm going to pretend I didn't hear that," and continued walking.

I came back forty-five minutes later. They'd set up a handwashing station with hand soap, hand sanitizer, and single-use gloves. The cigars were nowhere to be seen.

I gave them their permit and thanked them. But I didn't make any friends there. In fact, they threatened to call my boss. I told them I already had called him, which I had—after all, the guy who oversaw county inspections should be aware of what had been going on here. I have no patience with men like this. I say men because they were men—rude, arrogant, chauvinistic men.

Many years ago, there were even fewer women in my field than there are today, and sometimes I ran into conflicts. I live in an area where there aren't a tremendous number of women in positions of authority, and there still isn't much diversity, though things have come a long way.

A "Men's Club" in town, a well-established private organization hated by many local women, was on my list of facilities to inspect. The days I conducted those inspections were always an event, as the club did not permit women in the building. The only exceptions were escorts, and I certainly didn't fit that profile.

The organization was abuzz on those days I showed up, and I was definitely a thorn in their side. The men hated having to allow me in, so much so that they called my office to see if my employer could send a male inspector. Well, they were out of luck. I was the one and only.

I wasn't new to the type of treatment these gentlemen at the fishing rodeo and Men's Club displayed. But I was in charge, and while they didn't like it and were quick to tell me so, they had to listen to what I said. I was not interested in playing their games.

I recently experienced a situation with a male client that was more than a bit unnerving. This gentleman owed my company a lot of money and refused to pay the invoice, even though the government had reimbursed him for his purchased products. I am not talking small change; it came in around forty thousand dollars. We repeatedly sent invoices, made phone calls, and sent email and certified mail trying to collect the money.

We got no response, nothing.

Finally, he sent an email promising to pay by Friday. Friday came and went without payment or communication. He did the same a few weeks later, but no payment or further contact.

At this point, I was more than frustrated, so I began reaching out to authorities. It was a government contract and my reaching out to authorities really pissed him off. He told me he had never experienced such "aggressive and combative" behavior, and he threatened to sue me for defamation.

My point is that men aren't treated like this in the business world. As women, the expectation is that we will sit back and take whatever hand we are dealt. I have never heard a man who was defending himself called "aggressive and combative." I prefer the terms determined and persistent. I guess I should be happy he didn't lower himself to calling me a bitch, as is often done when women are assertive.

Though things have come a long way, it's not nearly far enough. I was really disappointed to learn that this attitude still existed in this day and age, as I hadn't experienced it in some time. I work in a male-dominated field, but I am fortunate to work with male colleagues who are professionals and know that we are all playing on the same ballfield.

Being a successful woman in business is not for the meek.

EIGHTEEN

Celebrity Chefs Are a Thorn in My Side

We've all watched one cooking show or another on television. At this point, there are more celebrity chefs than I can name. These shows drive me insane on multiple levels. Sure, the personalities are sometimes endearing, sometimes hysterical, and sometimes downright entertaining. But that's the point. *It's entertainment!*

I love some of these television personalities: Marcus Lemonis and his no-nonsense approach to business; Gordon Ramsey, who I think is hysterical; Robert Irvine was amazing; and who doesn't find Martha Stewart and Snoop Dog entertaining? But when it comes to television, entertainment and success don't equal safety.

I can assure you that what you see in front of the camera is not what happens in a "real" kitchen, and most people don't make that distinction.

Pick any one of those professional chefs, and I guarantee their staff follow the proper protocols when in the restaurants the chefs own and operate. They wash their hands with soap and water and properly dry them. They wear single-use gloves when working with ready-to-eat foods, and they restrain their hair (both the hair on their head and facial hair). They use thermometers to ensure they cook foods adequately. Yet to watch them on TV, you wouldn't know food safety protocols existed anywhere, ever, whether the person handling food is your favorite anchor from the morning news shows or a celebrity chef who knows better.

And as I travel and educate the masses, I hear it regularly.

The chefs stand at their workstations dressed to the nines. They can't put on hair nets or pull their hair up. It won't look good on TV. And there are some who wear more jewelry than I do on a typical business day.

I get it. They want to look nice.

The problem is, this is not what you should wear when you work in a commercial kitchen, and if someone represents themself as a chef, they should act like one.

After the TV personalities prepare a dish in the kitchen, the studio audience frequently samples the item. The audience at home doesn't realize that the food the audience is served was made in a commercial kitchen by cooks who followed guidelines set forth by the FDA Food Code. It's simply not necessary to clue them in to this fact.

Many years ago, I watched a daytime talk show host touch her face no less than ten times during one of her cooking segments. This is 100 percent a *great way to spread unwanted germs.*

There are multiple ways that producers could address these issues, if they chose to do so.

I thoroughly understand that there are time constraints, and to spend twenty to thirty seconds washing their hands every time it was warranted would be boring. To wash, rinse, and sanitize the countertop or cutting board would not make good TV. But I believe they have a responsibility to, at a minimum, acknowledge that these programs are for entertainment purposes only and tell people not to cook this way at home. Especially given that an estimated 1 in 6 Americans (or 48 million people) get sick every year, 128,000 are hospitalized, and 3,000 *die* from foodborne diseases.

There are multiple ways that producers could address these issues, if they chose to do so. I don't think it's intentional, and I don't believe they realize it's a problem, but I can assure you that most people in the foodservice industry believe it is, and we are very vocal about it.

The absence of any effort at food safety is unacceptable enough to most of us that we won't even watch this kind of programming unless we're doing so for research.

Social media videos have become a prevalent marketing mechanism, and they can work magnificently. However, the videos are often recorded in a working kitchen—and why wouldn't they be? I've seen some fantastic videos, but nothing makes me lose focus faster than a videographer and camera crew in a kitchen with their heads shoved up close and personal to a brick oven or a mouthwatering menu item while the employees work around them.

Why would I care?

Well, if a film crew or anyone else is working in a kitchen, they need to follow the same protocol as the employees working there, that's why.

Their hair falls out just like the employees' hair. It can end up in a customer's food just the same. I promise the customer will not give two hoots that it was someone on the film crew who shed the hair in their salad. It is just as disgusting. Marketing team members carry the same bacteria, and they should wash their hands, wear gloves, and follow the same protocol as the kitchen staff is required to as soon as they enter the kitchen—whether the staff is doing so or not.

While we all like to think our staff members are clean and not carrying any unwanted bacteria, outbreaks happen. If they use their cell phones to record videos, well, studies have shown that one in six cell phones have poop on them.

That's because nine out of ten people bring their smartphones into the bathroom with them. Charles Gerba, a famed University of Arizona microbiologist, found that cell phones carry ten times the bacteria of most toilet seats. Think about this the next time you see people using cell phones in a kitchen, or you use yours while you cook.

If these folks are going to work in kitchens, they must have some minimum food safety knowledge. Plus, operators really don't want them to post information that inadvertently goes against the current Food Code regulations. But I see this happen all the time in various types of marketing, not just videos.

I see Food Code faux pas on menu boards, websites, print materials, PDFs, videos—and it's not only in the images. It happens in the jargon, as well. Every time a "professional" marketer makes these errors, they cost a paying client business. It appears unprofessional, as though the client doesn't follow safety rules and regulations, which is off-putting to the consumer. My advice is to hire an expert to review marketing material after it is completed and before sending it off to your client. The extra effort in attention to detail will more than pay off in the end.

I always use national brands as an example.

Accuracy and attention to detail in food safety often equate to someone's life.

You never see Coca-Cola, Pepsi, Nike, UPS, FedEx, or McDonald's put errors in their advertising. Why? Because the ads are reviewed by many professionals, many times. It's called "branding." The ads are accurate and consistent. I'm referring to the colors they use, the font and the language they use, the style, the pictures, everything. I can't imagine McDonald's using an image of someone working in a kitchen that wasn't 100 percent accurate. It simply wouldn't happen. (And if it did, it would likely cost them a small fortune.)

Accuracy and attention to detail in food safety often equate to someone's life. If you are working in any facet of the industry, you are responsible for making damn sure you do things correctly.

NINETEEN

Do You Know What's Lurking in Your Kitchen?

Most of us would consider our kitchens to be the epitome of cleanliness, especially if you are like me. I call myself the Queen of Bleach because that's what I used to clean with when I was a kid and in my early years in the foodservice industry (bleach isn't permitted in most foodservice facilities anymore). That smell represents "clean" to me.

I used to scrub with bleach until my fingers were raw. I have ruined more clothes with bleach than you can imagine.

When the COVID-19 pandemic began in 2020, and you couldn't find bleach anywhere, I thought I was going to go nuts, and it had nothing to do with COVID. It was as if my number one cleaning supply was suddenly extinct.

Countertops, cupboards, stovetops, inside the refrigerator, the floor, the sinks, you name it—if the chemical won't ruin it, I'll wipe it down with bleach. Still, I know my kitchen is as laden with bacteria as anyone else's.

We recently purchased a new property and we haven't added a powder room on the lower level yet. So when people come in and need to wash their hands, they wash them in the kitchen sink. Doing this is a definite no-no, but hey, what do I know? It's likely not going to kill anyone, even though it's certainly not a best practice, and I am obsessive about cleaning the sink and everything around it. I am sure I do not have the only household where this occurs. Don't judge.

My point here is, every time someone washes their hands in the kitchen sink, all that elusive bacteria splashes around other things in the kitchen. It splashes onto clean dishes in the opposite sink (I can't be the only person who still hand-washes dishes), onto the counter, up into the aerator on the faucet (when did you last remove that and clean it?), and on anything else that happens to be within a few feet of the sink.

Moving right along, using the same knife, cutting board, and pair of gloves to slice the vegetables that you just used while chopping meat is an absolute no. Germs that can lead to foodborne illness due to cross-contamination are still something you must be thinking about when you're in your own kitchen.

It's best to have color-coded cutting boards when possible. Separate cutting boards for raw meat, poultry, and veggies. This way you minimize the risk of cross-contamination. High-density polyethylene (HDPE) are the most commonly used chopping boards in commercial kitchens because of their durability.

You don't want to inadvertently grab the gloves you used to clean the toilet when you prepare dinner!

Using the same pair of cleaning gloves over and over without cleaning the gloves themselves isn't ideal, either. It's best to switch out your gloves, properly get rid of the disposable type, and thoroughly clean your reusable cleaning gloves. I don't recommend you use the same kind of gloves for both cleaning and cooking at home, but if you do, at least use different colors. You don't want to inadvertently grab the gloves you used to clean the toilet when you prepare dinner! Yuck! I recommend using dedicated food service gloves for cooking.

There is no need to wash your poultry—chicken, turkey, duck. I don't care what your mother, father, grandma, aunt, or uncle did or said. Don't do it. It can do more harm than good.

The CDC says not to wash raw chicken. During washing, chicken juices can spread in the kitchen and contaminate other foods, utensils, and countertops. No one wants to spread any of the nastiness from raw chicken that we have discussed throughout this book just because you insist on washing it. Just be sure to cook it well.

Exception: Many years ago, my entire family was due at my mom's for Thanksgiving dinner. She expected many people, so she purchased a turkey that weighed at least thirty pounds, and she fully stuffed it with homemade dressing. It was common to stuff the turkey before cooking it thirty years ago. (I cannot imagine doing it today, not with what we know.) Anyway, Mom's kitchen was small. Several people had wandered through the kitchen throughout the morning.

At one point, my mother opened the oven door to baste the turkey, and let's say that oven rack was not made for a turkey that size. That bird came flying out of the oven like it was alive, slid its buttery self across the kitchen floor, and stopped against the opposite wall.

It was one of the funniest things I had ever seen. Fortunately, no one got burned, and only the turkey's pride was damaged.

But there was only one turkey, and everyone was expecting turkey for dinner. My mother's floor was not clean enough to eat off of, and I wanted no part of what was about to happen. She and my sister bathed that bird in the kitchen sink and put it back in the oven as if nothing had ever happened.

My own immediate family did not eat turkey that year. My daughter was barely older than a baby, and she still remembers the year the turkey slid across grandma's floor. Ugh!

Even back then, the cooked turkey was hot enough to reduce the bacteria that had collected on its outside to safe levels—until it skated across the kitchen floor. This incident created a whole new level of risk factors. God only knows what microorganisms may have been on the floor. Many people had walked through the kitchen, and there were pets.

We don't typically talk about the ridiculous things that happen, because we don't want anyone to judge. But we are all human and have "stories." It's important not to let them define us. Sometimes I shake my head thinking about it.

Sponges and cloth towels are the most frequently contaminated items in the kitchen. How many times have you used a dish towel to wipe off the counter after cooking, washed your hands, and then wiped your clean hands with that same towel? Use paper towels. It's one of the best ways to prevent cross-contamination.

Areas where food is stored or prepared have more bacteria and fecal contamination than other places in the home, according to a study by the National Sanitation Foundation (NSF). The NSF found that more than 75 percent of dish sponges and cloths have *Salmonella*, *E. coli*, and fecal matter on them, compared to 9 percent of bathroom faucet handles. Think about that.

Bacteria can be picked up by the dish sponges and cloths during the cleaning process—like when wiping up those icky messes such as blood from beef or poultry in kitchen sinks or on other surfaces. If not sanitized properly between uses, these items are a prime place for bacteria growth.

My mother-in-law used to get so upset with me because
I did not own a dish towel.

According to research, *Salmonella* grows on cloths stored overnight, even after being washed and rinsed in the sink. To reduce the risk of contamination, either strictly use paper towels, or use a new, clean cloth for each surface in your kitchen. Before using them again, be sure to wash your towels with bleach or other disinfectants.

If you hand-wash your dishes, allowing them to air dry on a clean dish rack is best practice so the dishware does not become contaminated with bacteria from dirty dishtowels. My mother-in-law used to get so upset with me because I did not own a dish towel. I had no need for them.

Typical bacteria found in the kitchen include *E. coli*, *Salmonella*, *Shigella*, *Campylobacter*, norovirus, and hepatitis A. *E. coli* can survive for hours on a surface, *Salmonella* can survive for about four hours, and hepatitis A can stay for months. You can lessen your chances of getting those germs in your mouth and nose by disinfecting each surface bacteria could have come into contact with, which means wiping down or spraying the surfaces in your kitchen where you've worked with food.

There are dozens of different kitchen utensils. It's important to be aware of how you use them and to safely care for them. Wash, rinse, and sanitize is standard protocol for all food contact surfaces.

When you use tongs or a fork to put raw meat or poultry on the grill, you must wash and sanitize them immediately afterward if you plan to use the same tools to serve the meal. And *do not* put cooked meat back on a plate it sat on before it was cooked!

The space we use to prepare meals for ourselves and our family is plagued with yeast, mold, and coliform bacteria...

Clean your utensils by hand-washing in hot, soapy water, rinsing, and then sanitizing them in a sanitizing solution. Make sure to air-dry them completely before putting them into the cupboard or, if you must, dry them with a single-use paper towel. Some other items that need frequent cleaning include cutting boards, coffee makers, the refrigerator—especially areas in contact with uncooked and unwashed food—and the kitchen sink and countertops.

Here is a frightening thought: the same NSF study I referenced above found that pet bowls are typically cleaner than coffee reservoirs, faucet handles, kitchen countertops, stove knobs, and cutting boards. Can you imagine eating from your pet's bowls? This study by one of the most trusted resources in the United States determined the bowls your pets use are cleaner than most of the areas in your kitchen. The space we use to prepare meals for ourselves and our family is plagued with yeast, mold, and coliform bacteria (a family of bacteria including *Salmonella* and *E. coli*).

Be aware of folks with food allergies. *Ask* when you invite guests if they have any food allergies, intolerances, or dietary restrictions. Check your ingredients carefully. The last thing you want at a gathering is someone dying because of a cross-contact issue with an allergen, or because you weren't aware Worcestershire sauce has anchovies in it, or because some barbecue sauces contain nuts.

When preparing food for an allergic individual, it is best to prepare their meal at a different time, in a different space, using different utensils. This is not the time for an "Oh, shit!" moment. Food allergies are no joke. They can be life-threatening, and the last thing you want to do is create a day of trauma for you and your guests.

TWENTY

The Farmer's Market Fiasco

We knew there were a million food safety issues at the most prominent local farmer's market in town. The market was open one day a week, and the vendors were in a large building. Everyone raved about the market and couldn't wait until the weekend arrived so they could visit and purchase their goods. Nothing could keep the locals away; they came rain, shine, sleet, or snow.

On Saturdays, local shoppers filled the building to capacity. They waited all week with anticipation to purchase their market goods. After all, *everyone* knows purchasing your food at a farmer's market is "much healthier" than buying it at the local grocery store!

> The person in charge of the health department had warned me that the building owner had neglected the facility for many years...

I am not one to prejudge anything or anyone, regardless of what I hear. My assistant and I went into the market prepared for anything, praying for the best. The person in charge of the health department had warned me that the building owner had neglected the facility for many years, and there were rumors of rodent issues.

As soon as we walked through the door, I saw a local farmer standing beside a skid of raw eggs—straight from his farm. Immediately,

I knew this was a problem. It was hot outside, there was no refrigeration to be seen, and the air conditioning in this building was non-existent.

Pennsylvania has precise requirements for selling farm-fresh eggs. And while some folks don't immediately place them in the refrigerator at home after collecting them from the nest, failure to do this is not permitted when selling them to the general public.

We introduced ourselves to the gentleman, who was shocked to see us. By now, we were used to that. It had become the typical reaction. I explained why we were there and what we'd be doing. I found a disposable cup and cracked two eggs into it to take their temperature.

We could already feel the tension in the building and see people in the crowd uneasily observing us. The day was not going to be easy. The vendors were not happy, and the locals didn't appear to be, either. It seemed they thought we were there to make trouble.

As the temperature on the thermometer continued to rise (as I was sure it would), I felt a sense of dread. I never like telling someone they have to shut down their business, let alone destroy their product. But if I had allowed him to keep the eggs, he would have brought them back into the building and begun selling them again as soon as we left. The only way to ensure this did not happen was to make him destroy them.

The building was hot—80°F to 85°F—and the eggs had been sitting on the floor (another issue) since early morning. And he had transported them in a vehicle that was not refrigerated. The eggs were way out of the safety range and had been for well over four hours, I was sure, based on the time the market opened.

I took the fact that this was his livelihood very seriously. I could tell by the various cartons, dates, and markings on the containers that he was reusing egg containers from the grocery store. I learned a long time ago that people are less than truthful to health inspectors, regardless of who they are, and if I didn't make him follow the guidelines, how would I handle the remaining fifty or so vendors in the building?

I watched as he threw the eggs in the dumpster and lost his entire day's sales. While I knew I was doing the right thing because I was responsible for the general public's health, inside, I was sick. There wasn't a person there who would have believed that, but it's true. The other vendors grew even more nervous and angry as their friend threw his day's income in the trash. The patrons were inquisitive, and the farmer's responses to them were vile and demeaning toward me.

All I could say was, "Unrefrigerated eggs are a threat to public health and it's important that everyone abide by the regulations. We are following the guidelines of the local jurisdiction. The report will be available on the Department of Ag website." It's challenging to find the right tone, but sometimes you need to explain your actions to the public, especially when you know you are right and protecting the very people who are upset with you.

Let's go back to some people not immediately refrigerating their farm eggs at home.

I know more than a few of you are thinking, "What the heck?" Much of the world doesn't refrigerate eggs. In many countries, you can find shelves of unrefrigerated, unwashed eggs right out in the open, waiting for customers to buy them.

Washing eggs gets rid of surface contaminants and provides a cleaner, fresher-looking egg.

But we can't do this in the United States. Here, we require suppliers to wash eggs before bringing them to outlets because of the bacteria that may live on the egg's shell. Washing eggs gets rid of surface contaminants and provides a cleaner, fresher-looking egg.

But, when the egg is washed, it removes a protective layer called the cuticle that coats the outside of the shell when a hen lays the egg in her nest. Removing this layer makes the egg more porous, reduces shelf life, and lets bacteria enter through the eggshell. Refrigerating eggs is therefore necessary to protect them after they're washed. It helps to prevent bacteria such as *Salmonella* from multiplying, and it maintains the quality of the egg.

At the farmer's market, tension continued to mount among vendors and customers. Let's just say the customers were not appreciative of my decisions. After the egg vendor incident, I inspected all vendors selling potentially hazardous foods (those that are temperature sensitive and must be controlled by maintaining specific temperature requirements) such as meats, cheeses, milk, or eggs. Of course, this made it appear that I was targeting specific vendors. While there is a certain truth to that, it's only because these were the most likely to make their customers ill.

The next vendor I inspected was across the aisle. She sold several items, and most of her food temperatures were within the guidelines. But not one of her products had a label showing the product's name; it's made-on, use-by, or sell-by date; or the initials of the person who made the food.

She argued that she knew exactly what every item was, when it was made, and who made it. While that may have been true, the inspection forms and the Food Code do not have guidelines with parameters stating "vendor knows exactly what the product is, when it was made, and by whom." The parameters are very black and white. The information needs to be recorded.

> She didn't want to hear anything I had to say,
> regardless of how I phrased it.

Her most serious violation was using dishwasher sanitizer in a three-bay sink to sanitize dishes and in sanitizing buckets for wiping counters. Dishwasher sanitizer is formulated differently from dish and counter sanitizer—it's toxic to humans and, unlike dish and counter sanitizers, dishwasher sanitizer must be washed off. But here she was, just pouring the sanitizer right onto the dishes in the sink that were going to air-dry...oh my God! Not to mention putting it right into the buckets she used to wipe things down. She didn't even have a dishwasher at this facility. It was a classic chemical contamination situation. But she didn't want to hear anything I had to say, regardless of how I phrased it.

Finally, after several minutes of politely trying to explain why she couldn't use sanitizer that way, I said, "If you don't get rid of it, you're going to kill someone. Dump it out now." She dumped it down the drain and got some of the proper sanitizer from one of the neighboring vendors. I fully believe in educating these individuals while I'm doing the inspections. I *want* them to learn and understand, so they don't repeat the behavior. Some don't care to hear it. This woman was one of them.

We continued through the building, encountering one violation after another. Vendors had to throw away more product, but the facilities remained open because they also sold acceptable items. Rumors went flying throughout the market, and vendors and stall owners moved quickly from one stand to another, pointing their fingers, speaking loudly, and staring at us. We were unwillingly on stage as we continued to move about, efficiently and effectively doing our job. It wasn't the first time we had been the victims of such hatred, and it wouldn't be the last.

We didn't realize it was going to get worse. Much, much, worse.

You wouldn't have known to look at us, but we were physically and emotionally exhausted. Several hours after we arrived, we were nearly back to where we'd started—only one or two more inspections to go.

One of our final stops was the meat counter. We approached an old-style meat cooler (it reminded me of my parents' coolers in our grocery store when I was a child in the late sixties and early seventies). I slid open the door and nearly gagged. Over the years, I have taught myself not to react like this, but an unmistakable stench hit me in the face.

The meat in this cooler was spoiled, and the vendor was actively selling it, a lot of it. At this point, this was the busiest vendor in the building. I quickly took a few temperatures to confirm they were inadequate and made sure nothing had spilled under the vents or somewhere else that might create such a putrid odor. Who knows, maybe there was a dead rat somewhere.

But upon rapid visual inspection, we didn't find anything else that could explain the odor. I was definitely smelling spoiled meat. I told the owner to stop selling the products. What ensued was like a scene from a movie that I did not want to be a part of.

As I spoke to the owner, who was being fully cooperative, I began to hear people angrily yelling from the other side of the counter. I turned around and saw sheer terror on my assistant's face. She looked like a deer caught in headlights. There were a lot of people on the other side of that counter, and they were *furious*. I asked my assistant to step back. She was in no way responsible for this.

This visual is priceless. My assistant was nearly six feet tall, and I am barely five foot one and weigh 110 pounds. I could barely see over the meat cooler. But I have a voice that projects nicely. I asked the people to please be quiet so I could explain what would happen. I was limited in the details I could provide, but they needed to know that dispersing was their best course of action. The meat counter would close and it would not reopen again that day.

One lady in particular asked obnoxious questions, hurled nasty comments, and didn't like any of my explanations. It seems this was the only day and the only location for her to purchase her meat—specifically bacon. I suggested many nearby solutions, and she found issues with all of them. The group grew, got more restless, and developed a mob mentality.

I stepped back to tell the owner quietly that he would have to take all of his meat products to the dumpster right outside and destroy them. This meant dumping bleach on the product. I had to be certain he couldn't dig it back out and sell it later. I needed to be sure no one would steal it from the dumpster and eat it. This product had all been well over 70°F for God knows how long.

I do not anger easily. If something makes me angry, the average person would have exploded much earlier. But when I get upset, there isn't much middle ground. I can go from zero to one hundred rapidly, and the lady who created this ever-growing mob was getting on my last nerve. There was no reasoning with her, and the crowd was beginning to threaten us physically.

It was unbelievable. Typically you can't tell which customers fall into the high-risk category, meaning they are at a higher risk of getting a foodborne illness than most. But I assure you that everyone in this mob was in that group that day. That meat might not only have made them sick; it could have given them an illness with lifelong ramifications or killed them.

The mob leader wanted a slab of bacon. I am not a violent person, but I wanted to throw that slab of bacon at her and shout, "Go ahead and eat that seventy-degree bacon, b****!"

I was beyond frustrated and angry with these people. They would not listen to explanation or reason, nor be quiet long enough for me to tell them the importance of my inspection. I, of course, would *never* do such a thing, but it had been a very long, hard, frustrating day, and it was one time in my life when I felt like saying, "If you don't think I know what I'm talking about, go ahead and eat it."

We had a direct line to the police department so we wouldn't tie up the emergency operator by calling 911 if we needed help. As the very people we were trying to protect continued to verbally and physically threaten us, I glanced around and told my assistant to very discreetly call that line. We needed a police escort to get out of the building.

These vendors weren't accustomed to being inspected
or to following guidelines.

We had the police on speed dial, and they knew we only called when we had a true emergency. They arrived in a matter of minutes. The mob calmed down and dispersed as soon as the police got there. The crowd was pretty surprised, actually, when the police showed up, especially considering the officers knew us and were in total support of our efforts. Whatever credibility they assumed we lacked was immediately resurrected.

I blame events of that day on the lack of leadership in the health department during the several years before my tenure. These vendors weren't accustomed to being inspected or to following guidelines. Suddenly a health inspector—a woman, at that—showed up and enforced the Food Code. Even though I began as softly as possible, there were so many severe violations that it seemed I was being unduly harsh.

As we left the building with our police escort, I laughed and said to my assistant, "One day, I will write a book about this fiasco and the bizarre experiences I've had as a health inspector." We all laughed as we got in our various vehicles to leave the market.

As we pulled out of the parking lot, I noticed that a small market was open across the street. So I said, "Hey, let's go over there and get that one out of the way."

You would have thought I'd have had enough for the day, but no, not me. Just. One. More. It was a small market, and it wouldn't take long.

We parked the car out front and went into the market. The look of shock is always a little bit funny, only because it's as if these people have never heard of a health inspector. I do get the shock factor of it being a Saturday, too. Not many health inspectors are out and about on Saturdays.

What was it with people and eggs that day?

We headed back to the walk-in cooler, and on the way, we walked past several cases of eggs sitting out on the floor. The owner assured me they were recently delivered, but I felt the boxes and they were at room temperature, so I knew she was lying to me. I asked her to get me the invoice. The invoice was dated two days prior. Now I knew I couldn't trust her. What was it with people and eggs that day?

I opened the walk-in cooler door, and as I entered, I saw four hog heads—yes, heads—sitting on the bottom shelf, immediately over produce on the floor. They had placed the hog heads directly on the shelf, so if anything dripped (and it did), it landed on the lettuce, lemons, and limes underneath.

I want to tell you this was all I saw, but it wasn't. Directly at the back of the cooler were halves of beef hanging there like in a butcher shop. I've seen hog heads and beef carcasses before, but in the appropriate environment, and this was not it. Not to mention all the ready-to-eat foods and fresh produce dispersed among the freshly cut raw meat. This cooler was a disaster. Why did I think this would be easy? Just. One. More.

When we finally left the facility, a lady stood in the doorway of the apartment next door. She was selling burritos and water out of a cooler. Selling anything out of a cooler in one's doorway is neither legal nor safe. We walked over and asked to see her permit, knowing full well she didn't have one.

I took a few temperatures that were well below the minimum hot-food holding temperature of 140°F. I was very kindly and empathetically explaining to her that she was not permitted to sell her products, especially on the doorstep of her apartment building, when her burly husband emerged and threatened me. He told the woman she should continue selling the burritos and water.

I had already seen "her" ID and knew it was a fake. My guess was that something was going on besides the illegal sale of burritos.

As the burly man continued to yell and physically threaten her and us, and he wouldn't let her take the burritos away, we had to make our second call of the day to the local police department. It turned out the police were familiar with the burrito lady and her burly husband.

It was time for us to go home. Mental note: Never assume anything is going to be easy.

TWENTY-ONE

Only a Stepping Stone

I only intended to be a health inspector for a year. It was intended as a stepping stone for me. But as it turned out, I was a health inspector for three years. It felt good when I left, and things had turned around. I felt better about the public health situation. I wasn't closing as many restaurants, and most of the facilities that had flown under the radar for years had cleaned up their act substantially.

In my first year, I closed 20 percent of the restaurants in the city. That did not go over well with anyone, including the borough council. Due to the number of closures and the community backlash, the borough council required me to present precisely why this occurred. I understood their position entirely.

I wish you could have seen their faces when I began showing slides of mold in ice machines...

Before me, there hadn't been an issue. Why would there be? No one had been doing inspections. Most of the documentation was fraudulent. Of course, the council didn't realize this was the case. I wish you could have seen their faces when I began showing slides of mold in ice machines that you could scoop out with your hands, cockroaches nesting inside equipment, employees washing dishes in mop sinks, case upon case of chicken thawing in filthy kitchen sinks beside clean dishes that were air drying on the drain board, fresh duck in a freezer (feathers still intact), carp being sold out the back doors of restaurants, and the disreputable kitchen of the fine dining establishment they all ate at regularly.

Yes, to their surprise, this all happened in their beloved small town, right under their noses.

Council meetings were advertised and public. Every nemesis I had within my jurisdiction showed up. They'd all called the borough office and the health department to complain about the new health inspector—regularly. Every time I closed a restaurant, the closure sign that we posted on the door was plastered all over Facebook before I could pull out of the parking lot. Once, I was met by a reporter on my way in the door to conduct a reinspection.

The public appetite for this was insatiable.

> Owners of many of the sites were in the audience waiting
> to slander my character.

As I was giving the council my presentation, I showed the images and explained the risks involved with each photo: hepatitis A, *E. coli*, norovirus, *Staphylococcus aureus*, nontyphoidal *Salmonella*, *Salmonella* Typhi, and more. Owners of many of the sites were in the audience waiting to slander my character. Members of the town council watched with absolute horror—several were doctors and lawyers—and they understood what they learned from me. I asked them if they or their families dined at these locations. Pictures speak a thousand words, and these were graphic. When I completed my presentation, there wasn't much room for public comment. I answered all of the council's questions.

I was articulate, confident, and well prepared. I walked out with my head held high. But I knew winning this battle placed me in a precarious situation. I had a permit to carry a concealed weapon by then, and I took advantage of it. It made me feel safer as I walked into the dark parking lot alone after the meeting. Fortunately, no one put me in a situation where I needed to protect myself.

Over the next few years, I learned from my stores, and they learned from me. I held classes at the local community center for those who wanted to know more. Some were like sponges, wanting to learn as much as I could teach them. I even gave a few my cell number to field questions when they ran into a problem trying to sort things out to reopen after being shut down. I was always willing to help those who were ready to learn.

At the end of my tenure in the position, I'd enter facilities to inspect and there wasn't as much hatred as there had been three years prior. Most operators had come to respect me and the position I held. There were still a few holdouts, but when you're in a position of authority, it's to be expected—it's how life works. I'm okay with it. I know I made a difference. It felt good to know that I had potentially saved dozens, if not hundreds, of lives in those three years. I am proud of what I accomplished and my stepping stone became a rewarding building block.

All these years later, I still get phone calls every now and then from someone asking a question or just saying hi. That gives me a sense of accomplishment.

About three years ago, one of these restaurants called to tell me that the town council was revamping standards and hiring new health inspectors. Was I interested in returning? When I did inspections, we had nearly three hundred facilities to inspect twice a year and had to handle complaints, emergencies, and reinspections. And I was the only inspector.

It was nearly impossible. I did inspections on evenings and weekends, too, which I believe should happen anyway, to avoid missing something important that might occur. Imagine the response I got to that!

Since that time, many new restaurants have opened and new operations have moved into the area. I was happy to hear they were hiring additional inspectors and someone new would be in charge of the program. However, I had no interest in taking part. While I appreciated the suggestion, I had moved on to new food safety adventures.

On occasion, when I'm searching for something on my computer, doing research, or writing an article, I come across some of the more horrific images that I took during inspections. It takes me right back to those moments in time. I can see the surroundings, hear the sounds, and smell the odors from the very day. The image of the hooved legs dangling over the edge of the cardboard box in the freezer is cringe-worthy, and the photograph of the thermometer in the rotten bacon at the farmer's market makes me wrinkle my nose at the thought of the putrid smell. The images of the violations from the Chinese restaurant with mounds of raw chicken thawing in the sink and dead cockroaches piled in the corners while employees washed dishes in the mop sink are detailed, vivid flashbacks scorched into my memory. My experiences in the role were both meaningful and impactful for me. I never dreamed I would see the things I saw or had the experiences I had during those three years. Sometimes I feel like it was a dream. But then I look in my wallet and realize I still have my permit to carry, and I still own that handgun.

It wasn't a dream, though some moments were a nightmare.

TWENTY-TWO

I Don't Want My Food Where My Dirty Underwear's Been

Frank Yiannis, former Deputy Commissioner of Food Policy and Response at the Food and Drug Administration, has said many times, "The goal of the food safety professional should be to create a *food safety culture*, not a food safety program." This statement could not be more accurate. You can have the best food safety program in the world. Still, if the people within the industry that created the program are not following guidelines, the plan is not worth the paper it's written on. The likelihood of a foodborne illness catastrophe is high.

Our food safety standards begin at home, when we are young. Basic rules include:

- *Keep your hands clean* by washing them often in soapy water and by not licking your fingers while preparing food.
- Separate raw and cooked foods.
- Cook food to the proper temperature.
- Be careful about cross-contamination.
- Don't put cooked foods on platters that hold raw food you still need to cook.

When I think back to my own childhood and what I witnessed from my mom and grandparents, I sometimes wonder how I lived. Even realizing that many things have changed since then, including processing habits and the fact that the bacteria we deal with today wasn't as prevalent back then, I know I still survived some pretty scary food safety habits.

As I mentioned before, I grew up in rural America, where pastoral thoughts and habits abound. My grandmothers each had the "old-time" crocks always on top of their stoves. They both used these to hold leftover grease from bacon, pork chops, hamburger—whatever meat they happened to make. They would use the drippings from cooking meat to fry eggs, potatoes, or anything else that needed some oil in the pan.

I never once saw either one of them empty the crock to clean it. They made the best fried potatoes and fried green tomatoes I've eaten to this day. But I bet the lard on the bottom of those crocks was older than I was.

Essentially if there was ground beef in the kitchen, she ate it raw.

My mom's family was from the South, and she deep-fried *everything*. We lived in an old house with lath and plaster walls. The kitchen had a built-in cupboard, and you could see the strips of wood in the wall at the back of our floor-to-ceiling pantry. Mom had a brown paper bag—like a lunch bag—she kept on the top shelf, filled with flour, seasoning salt, and pepper. Regardless of what she fried, we got the brown bag out of the cupboard and shook the food in that mixture to coat it with seasoning before placing it in the hot oil. Then we put the bag back on the shelf in the cupboard. We used that seasoning for fish, pork, tenderloin, and chicken. The same seasoning, in the same bag. I shake my head thinking about it.

I remember Mom eating some of the raw ground beef mixture every time she made meatloaf, meatballs, or hamburgers. Essentially if there was ground beef in the kitchen, she ate it raw. We grew up eating rare hamburgers—I'm talking blood-soaked-bun rare. Keep in mind that until the 1993 Jack in the Box *E. coli* outbreak—when the *Escherichia coli* O157:H7 bacterium infected 732 people and killed 4 children—no one thought this was a problem.

We had a large family, and many people were at our home every Thanksgiving. The turkey was always massive, usually too large to fit in the refrigerator with all of the other side dishes that we prepared. I vividly remember Mom stuffing our bird with dressing around midnight or so on Thanksgiving Eve and letting it sit out on the side of the old wood and gas cook stove until five in the morning, when she'd get up and put it in the oven.

Often, it had been out thawing in the kitchen sink before all this, too. We always had something thawing on the counter or in the sink. I got the "flu" after more than one Thanksgiving dinner. Looking back, I'm pretty sure it was food poisoning. I couldn't eat cherry pie, one of my favorites, for years due to an epic case of the "Thanksgiving flu" that ruined it for me.

Over the years, I traveled to many locations and heard story after story about unsafe food preparation practices. I don't have a natural poker face, never have. Whatever I am thinking is usually written all over my face like chalk on a chalkboard. As a conference leader or presenter to a large group of people, sometimes I hear shared stories. Shocking stories. But it's a mark of professionalism to keep personal reactions under wraps. If the person on stage reacts too negatively to what people in the audience share, regardless of what it is, it won't be long before the group stops interacting. That's the last thing a presenter wants. So I have really had to focus on controlling my body language and facial expressions.

Some comments, I will never forget. I would love to tell you they're somehow geographically or demographically isolated, but that's not true. We can find a fundamental lack of food safety knowledge across the board. I've had people tell me they wrapped their frozen turkey in an electric blanket to thaw it (say what?). Someone else said they put their turkey in the dryer to defrost. I can barely take hearing a pair of tennis shoes pounding the sides of my own dryer, let alone a twenty-pound turkey. And this was before we had shelves in our dryers to place sweaters and sneakers on—so that turkey was tumbling! Can you imagine how bruised that bird was when it finished?!

And then there was the woman who washed her collard greens in the washing machine. I don't know about you, but I don't want my food anywhere my dirty underwear has been!

Poaching fish in the dishwasher while washing dishes—or any time—is not a good idea, either.

The absolute worst thing anyone ever told me came from a young man in one teaching session who said he was mad at his shop owner, so he urinated in a bucket of sauce. Did he say it to get a reaction, or was it true? I don't know, but what I do know is, by the end of the day, he was out of the group, his boss had police interviewing him, and he was unemployed. Tampering with food is something you never joke about. It's a felony.

TWENTY-THREE

This Is Me!

Thank you for taking this time to read about my experiences. I wrote this book with humor—it's who I am—but that doesn't negate the seriousness of the subject matter. If you don't take anything else away from reading this, please understand that foodborne illnesses are 100 percent preventable, and no one should ever die from eating food. No one.

As I wrote this, it brought back a barrage of memories, some very fond memories of people who have mentored and coached me along the way, and many memories of hysterical moments that happened over the years. Not to mention thoughts of the friends I've made and the friends I've lost. Tragedies and triumphs.

The hours I spent digging through my memory bank dredged up more unhappy memories of childhood trauma than I care to remember, too. It took a long time to get where I am today. Those wounds don't magically disappear. It takes a lot of work, and typically we do it without much of a support system because mental health isn't something we frequently discuss.

That reality needs to change. Trauma follows us throughout our lives, in one aspect or another, and it rears its ugly head when we least expect it. I can tell you this: it took years for me to accept who I am and know that nothing is wrong with me.

On that note, when the song "This Is Me" was released as part of *The Greatest Showman* soundtrack, I listened to the lyrics, and I cried.

Now that you've finished reading *Who Watches the Kitchen,*
I'd love to hear what you thought of it! By reviewing this book
on the Amazon and Goodreads listings, you help other readers
determine if this is the best book for them.

Acknowledgments

Where do I begin? I would be remiss if I did not start with my husband. We had been married six months the day I called him and said, "I quit my job."

It wasn't just a job; this was a job that I loved, and I happened to earn a good living while working there. And I was our primary source of income.

It only took a second, but as soon as he realized I was serious, he said, "It'll be okay." I will never forget that moment. It was the first time in my life I had ever felt that unconditional support. There was no backup plan. I had had no intention of quitting. I didn't aspire to start my own business.

Six months later, I decided that was exactly what I would do. It has not been easy. Being an entrepreneur is the bumpiest roller coaster ride you will ever get on (no one ever tells you that part of the story), but it is also the most rewarding. Eleven years later, my husband is still my biggest supporter, even on the worst days. I couldn't accomplish half of what I do without him. So thank you, Tim, for your unconditional love and support for the past twenty years. I love you more than you know.

I want to thank my children, Ashley and Jeffrey. I love them to the moon and back and more. Their families are a gift for which I am beyond grateful.

Melissa, you show up every day to support me through the good, the bad, and the ugly on this entrepreneurial journey. Thank you for your unwavering support and commitment.

This book wouldn't be possible without so many others.

Adrienne, you helped me get published in my first publication, and I'm still writing, 300+ articles later.

Matt Regusci, thank you for being a friend. I think there's a sitcom in that somewhere. Seriously, who would have thought a LinkedIn contact would have turned into such a remarkable friendship and turned out such great work and a podcast. Thank you for your kindness, support, honesty, and laughs!

Thank you to all the individuals who believed in me and gave me an opportunity along the way: Bill, who hired me and allowed me to keep my job even though I wasn't old enough to work. Without him, I don't know where my life would have gone. Donna, who promoted me twice even though the odds were not in my favor. Kirk, who recommended me for a promotion even though I was young and not a likely candidate.

Many others worked with me and supported me along my journey. Thank you all, especially those brave enough to be with me during those bizarre inspection investigations—you know who you are. Your support is appreciated.

Darin Detwiler and Hal King have inspired me in various ways during my career. Thank you for the fantastic work you do to educate the world about food safety. The commitment and dedication you gentlemen have to this mission are paramount. You have each impacted the lives of so many that I'm sure you don't even realize. The work you have done will continue to impact lives around the globe for years to come. Folks starting out in the food safety world aspire to follow your lead.

Francine Sinclair, thank you for so many great introductions and so much social media assistance! Without you, I would not have met Paula, who was instrumental in writing this book. You are a matchmaker from heaven.

Paula Diaco, I have so enjoyed this process. Your insight and assistance have been inspirational, and I couldn't have written this book without you.

I am already looking forward to writing the next one.

Resources

Learn everything you've ever wanted to know about the food supply chain but were too afraid to ask — plus a lot you never wanted to know and will regret learning in Francine's highly-rated podcast, *Don't Eat POOP!* She and her co-host Matthew Regusci keep the material funny, fresh, and served every Tuesday.

Stay up-to-date on all food safety news, and FDA recalls at https://savvyfs.com/food-safety-news/

Organization and Professional Resources

As one of the top experts in her field, Francine Shaw helps businesses make SMART. SAFE. SAVVY.™ decisions in food safety education, compliance, and regulation through products, services, and training.

Speaking

Francine Shaw is a sought-after motivational speaker for entrepreneurs, high-performing professionals, and women's organizations, where she inspires and motivates. Her insights, strategies, and expertise unlock success for business and personal growth while igniting her attendee's drive to succeed. She is on a mission to see women take their place in all male-dominated industries.

Industry Events

Francine Shaw, CP-FS, CFSM, FSP, FMP, has had the pleasure of helping numerous clients around the world. Some of the organizations she has spoken for include the National Environmental Health

Association, Association of Nutrition of Foodservice Professionals, School Nutrition Association, and ISSA/INTERCLEAN. Her impressive roster of clients also includes companies like McDonald's, Subway, Marriott, Domino's, Paradies Lagardere, Diversey, and others.

Discuss your event with Francine by booking a call at her site: https://savvyfs.com/speaking/#event

My Trusted Source

A business solution should be easy-to-use, reduce liabilities, eliminate the middleman, and have no transaction costs. My Trusted Source facilitates the connection between consumers, buyers, suppliers, and service providers to connect all aspects of the supply chain while improving transparency, traceability, and efficiency.

To see how you can save money and time, visit https://www.my-trustedsc.com/

TracSavvy

Francine's decades in foodservice give her an advantage in understanding your struggles in maintaining compliance and training standards. Both are imperative to your company's success. With TracSavvy, you reduce the risk of health code violations and streamline certifications. Automated notifications, tracking, and data all in one place.

To find out more information, visit https://savvyfs.com/tracsavvy/

Addition Resources

To keep it savvy with your customers, staff, and bottom line Francine also offers the additional resources below.

Audits

Internal Audits

Training

Haccp (international haccp alliance)

Advanced Training
Certified HACCP Lead Instructor

Additional services
Curriculum Development
Food Safety/HACCP plan development
Subject Matter Expert Services
Supply Chain Verification
Food Safety Training Program Development
S.O.P. Program Development

Francine L. Shaw is a dynamic and driven business leader with a passion for innovation and success. As the founder and CEO of Savvy Food Safety and Co-Founder of My Trusted Source, she is committed to pushing the boundaries and constantly evolving in the ever-changing landscape of the foodservice industry from one end of the supply chain to the other. With a proven track record of driving growth and achieving objectives, she leads and inspires others to reach their full potential.

https://savvyfs.com/

X @FSTS3787
Instagram and Facebook @savvyfoodsafety
LinkedIn @https://www.linkedin.com/in/francinelshaw/

Sources

Prologue

Centers for Disease Control and Prevention. "Estimates of Foodborne Illness in the United States." Last reviewed November 5, 2018. https://www.cdc.gov/foodborneburden/index.html.

World Health Organization. "Food Safety." Posted May 19, 2022. https://www.who.int/news-room/fact-sheets/detail/food-safety.

Chapter 5

Berfield, Susan. "Inside Chipotle's Contamination Crisis." *Bloomberg*, December 22, 2015. https://www.bloomberg.com/features/2015-chipotle-food-safety-crisis/.

Centers for Disease Control and Prevention. "Norovirus Burden and Trends." Last reviewed May 8, 2023. https://www.cdc.gov/norovirus/trends-outbreaks/burden-US.html.

Coleman, Kejuan. "Crisis Management – Chipotle Case Study." *Kejuan Coleman's Blog*, February 20, 2019. https://kejuandot.wordpress.com/2019/02/20/crisis-management-chipotle-case-study/.

Chapter 5, *continued*

Cooper, Kindra. "How Chipotle Regained Customer Trust After the E. Coli Outbreak in 2015." *Customer Contact Week Digital*, October 16, 2019. https://www.customercontactweekdigital.com/performance-metrics/articles/chipotle-behind-the-foil.

Gillespie, Patrick. "Chipotle's stock falls after E. coli scare." *CNN Business*, November 2, 2015. https://money.cnn.com/2015/11/02/investing/chipotle-stock-falls-after-e-coli-outbreak/.

ImperialDade. "Hand Dryers vs Paper Towels: 6 Reasons Paper Towels are the Best Choice." *Imperial Dade Insights*, May 21, 2020. https://www.imperialdade.com/blog/hand-dryers-vs-paper-towels.

Kilgore, Tomi. "Chipotle's stock suffers biggest loss of the year after sales warning." *Marketwatch.com*, June 20, 2017. https://www.marketwatch.com/story/chipotles-stock-tumbles-as-sales-warning-prompts-target-cuts-2017-06-20.

Kimmitt, P. T. and K. F. Redway. "Evaluation of the potential for virus dispersal during hand drying: a comparison of three methods." *Journal of Applied Microbiology*, 120, no. 2 (February 2016): 478–486. https://doi.org/10.1111/jam.13014.

Kirshner-Breen, Stanley. "Chipotle Attempts to Recover From E. Coli PR Disaster: A Case Study." *Medium*, August 3, 2017. https://medium.com/@kbreenconsulting/chipotle-attempts-to-recover-from-e-coli-pr-disaster-a-case-study-1023a31f29b0.

Marler, Bill. "Chipotle Mexican Grill Agrees to Pay $25 Million Fine and Enter a Deferred Prosecution Agreement to Resolve Charges Related to Foodborne Illness Outbreaks." *Marler Blog*, April 21, 2020. https://www.marlerblog.com/?s=chipotle.

Chapter 5, *continued*

News Desk. "Chipotle agrees to pay $25 million federal fine for role in some outbreaks." *Food Safety News*, April 22, 2020. https://www.foodsafetynews.com/2020/04/chipotle-agrees-to-pay-25-million-federal-fine-for-role-in-some-outbreaks/.

Ortiz, Aimee. "Chipotle to Pay $25 Million Fine for Tainted Food." *The New York Times*, April 21, 2020. https://www.nytimes.com/2020/04/21/business/chipotle-tainted-food-settlement.html.

Platt, Frances Marion. "Class action settlement announced in Mohonk Mountain House norovirus lawsuit." *Hudson Valley One*, April 19, 2016. https://hudsonvalleyone.com/2016/02/06/class-action-settlement-announced-in-mohonk-mountain-house-norovirus-lawsuit/.

Polansek, Tom. "Chipotle settles sick customers' claims, avoiding court battles." *Reuters*, September 8, 2016. https://www.reuters.com/article/us-chipotle-settlements-idUSKCN11E30I.

Prisco, Joanna. "Norovirus Shuts Down Historic New York State Resort." *ABC News*, February 10, 2014. https://abcnews.go.com/Travel/virus-shuts-historic-york-state-resort/story?id=22446268.

The Marler Clark Network. Foodborne Illness Outbreak Database. http://outbreakdatabase.com/.

U.S. Food & Drug Administration. "Chipotle Mexican Grill Agrees to Pay $25 Million Fine to Resolve Charges Stemming from More Than 1,100 Cases of Foodborne Illness." April 21, 2020. https://www.fda.gov/inspections-compliance-enforcement-and-criminal-investigations/press-releases/chipotle-mexican-grill-agrees-pay-25-million-fine-resolve-charges-stemming-more-1100-cases-foodborne.

Chapter 6

Abend, Lisa. "When the World's Top Restaurant Serves Up a Bug." *TIME Magazine*, March 10, 2013. https://world.time.com/2013/03/10/when-the-worlds-top-restaurant-serves-up-a-bug/.

Bartsch, Sarah M., Lindsey Asti, Sindiso Nyathi, Marie L. Spiker, Bruce Y. Lee. "Estimated Cost to a Restaurant of a Foodborne Illness Outbreak." *Sage Journals* 133, no. 3 (April 15, 2018): 274–286. https://doi.org/10.1177/0033354917751129.

Centers for Disease Control and Prevention. "List of Multistate Foodborne Outbreak Notices." Last reviewed June 13, 2023. https://www.cdc.gov/foodsafety/outbreaks/multistate-outbreaks/outbreaks-list.html.

Centers for Disease Control and Prevention. "E. coli Outbreak Linked to Packaged Salads." Food Safety Alert, March 3, 2022. https://www.cdc.gov/ecoli/2021/o157h7-12-21/index.html.

Centers for Disease Control and Prevention. "Listeria Outbreak Linked to Packaged Salads Produced by Fresh Express." Food Safety Alert, March 8, 2022. https://www.cdc.gov/listeria/outbreaks/packaged-salad-12-21-b/index.html.

Centers for Disease Control and Prevention. "Listeria Outbreak Linked to Packaged Salads Produced by Dole." Food Safety Alert, April 4, 2022. https://www.cdc.gov/listeria/outbreaks/packaged-salad-mix-12-21/index.html.

Centers for Disease Control and Prevention. "E. coli Outbreak Linked to Baby Spinach." Food Safety Alert, January 6, 2022. https://www.cdc.gov/ecoli/2021/o157h7-11-21/index.html.

Chapter 6, *continued*

Centers for Disease Control and Prevention. "Salmonella Outbreak Linked to Salami Sticks." Food Safety Alert, December 8, 2021. https://www.cdc.gov/salmonella/i45-10-21/index.html.

Centers for Disease Control and Prevention. "Salmonella Outbreak Linked to Seafood." Food Safety Alert, December 6, 2021. https://www.cdc.gov/salmonella/thompson-10-21/index.html.

Centers for Disease Control and Prevention. "Salmonella Outbreak Linked to Onions." Food Safety Alert, February 2, 2022. https://www.cdc.gov/salmonella/oranienburg-09-21/index.html.

Centers for Disease Control and Prevention. "Salmonella Outbreak Linked to Italian-Style Meats." Food Safety Alert, October 26, 2021. https://www.cdc.gov/salmonella/italian-style-meat-08-21/index.html.

Centers for Disease Control and Prevention. "E. coli Outbreak Linked to Cake Mix." Investigation Notice, September 16, 2021. https://www.cdc.gov/ecoli/2021/o121-07-21/index.html.

Centers for Disease Control and Prevention. "Salmonella Outbreak Linked to BrightFarms Packaged Salad Greens." Food Safety Alert, October 6, 2021. https://www.cdc.gov/salmonella/typhimurium-07-21/index.html.

Centers for Disease Control and Prevention. "Listeria Outbreak Linked to Fully Cooked Chicken." Food Safety Alert, September 10, 2021. https://www.cdc.gov/listeria/outbreaks/precooked-chicken-07-21/index.html.

Chapter 6, *continued*

Centers for Disease Control and Prevention. "Salmonella Outbreak Linked to Frozen Cooked Shrimp." Food Safety Alert, September 21, 2021. https://www.cdc.gov/salmonella/weltevreden-06-21/index.html.

Centers for Disease Control and Prevention. "Salmonella Outbreak Linked to Raw Frozen Breaded Stuffed Chicken Products." Food Safety Alert, October 13, 2021. https://www.cdc.gov/salmonella/enteritidis-06-21/index.html.

Centers for Disease Control and Prevention. "Salmonella Outbreak Linked to Jule's Cashew Brie." Food Safety Alert, July 7, 2021. https://www.cdc.gov/salmonella/duisburg-04-21/index.html.

Centers for Disease Control and Prevention. "Salmonella Outbreak Linked to Ground Turkey." Food Safety Alert, May 18, 2021. https://www.cdc.gov/salmonella/hadar-04-21/index.html.

Centers for Disease Control and Prevention. "Listeria Outbreak Linked to Queso Fresco Made by El Abuelito Cheese Inc." Food Safety Alert, May 14, 2021. https://www.cdc.gov/listeria/outbreaks/hispanic-soft-cheese-02-21/index.html.

Centers for Disease Control and Prevention. "E. coli Outbreak with Unknown Food Source." Investigation Notice, March 11, 2021. https://www.cdc.gov/ecoli/2021/o157h7-02-21/index.html.

Chang, David and Deanna Durante. "Officials Confirm 3rd Death in Montco Hepatitis A Outbreak, Restaurant Reopens." *NBC News*, January 20, 2022. https://www.nbcphiladelphia.com/news/health/officials-confirm-3rd-death-in-montco-hepatitis-a-outbreak-restaurant-reopens/3113717/.

Chapter 6, *continued*

Chappell, Bill. "'World's Best Restaurant' Blamed For Diners' Illnesses." *NPR*, March 8, 2013. https://www.npr.org/sections/thetwo-way/2013/03/08/173847217/worlds-best-restaurant-blamed-for-diners-illnesses.

Kowitt, Beth. "Why Our Food Keeps Making Us Sick." *Fortune Magazine*, May 6, 2016. https://fortune.com/longform/food-contamination/.

Chapter 11

Animal Rescue Professionals Association. "Rats Create How Many Relatives In 18 Months?" *Animal Rescue Professionals Association Blog*, June 10, 2019. https://www.animalrescueprofessionals.org/animal-facts/rats-breed-so-quickly/.

Rentokil. "How quickly can rats multiply in your facility?" *Rentokil Blog*, October 29, 2018. https://www.rentokil.com/us/blog/quickly-can-rats-multiply-facility/.

Smithsonian's National Zoo & Conservation Biology Institute. "Norway Rat." Norway Rat. Accessed June 29, 2023. https://nationalzoo.si.edu/animals/norway-rat.

Chapter 13

Centers for Disease Control and Prevention. "Estimates of Foodborne Illness in the United States." Last reviewed November 5, 2018. https://www.cdc.gov/foodborneburden/index.html.

Chapter 18

Cardenas, Edward. "Study: 9 Out Of 10 People Use Their Cell Phone In The Bathroom." CBS News, June 30, 2015. https://www.cbsnews.com/detroit/news/study-9-out-of-10-people-use-their-cellular-phone-in-the-bathroom/.

Centers for Disease Control and Prevention. "Estimates of Foodborne Illness in the United States." Last reviewed November 5, 2018. https://www.cdc.gov/foodborneburden/index.html.

Matthews, Susan E. "Why your cellphone has more germs than a toilet." *Today Health*, August 30, 2012.

Song, Sora. "Study: 1 in 6 Cell Phones Contaminated With Fecal Matter." *TIME Magazine*, October 17, 2011. https://healthland.time.com/2011/10/17/study-1-in-6-cell-phones-contaminated-with-fecal-matter/.

Chapter 19

Centers for Disease Control and Prevention. "Chicken and Food Poisoning." Last reviewed October 31, 2022. https://www.cdc.gov/foodsafety/chicken.html.

Healthline. "The 9 Dirtiest Spots in Your Home." *Healthline*, updated April 27, 2020. https://www.healthline.com/health/germy-places.

National Sanitation Foundation. "Clean the Germiest Home Items." NSF, February 2021. https://www.nsf.org/blog/consumer/clean-germiest-home-items.

Chapter 19, *continued*

NSF International. "2011 NSF International Household Germ Study." NSF International, 2011. https://d2evkimvhatqav.cloudfront. net/documents/2011_NSF_Household_Germ_Study_exec-summary.pdf?v=1594928300.

Chapter 22

Yiannis, Frank. Retrieved February 11, 2022. LinkedIn. https://www. linkedin.com/feed/update/urn:li:activity:6895732799853137921/.

www.ingramcontent.com/pod-product-compliance
Lightning Source LLC
Chambersburg PA
CBHW060533130626
46553CB00002B/728